تهران ۱۹۸۰

محمد باقر افخمی
محمد

A Country Doctor's
COMMON SENSE HEALTH MANUAL

Other Books by the Same Author

Doctor Hurdle's Program to Retain Youthfulness
Low Blood Sugar: A Doctor's Guide to Its Effective Control

J. Frank Hurdle, M.D.

A Country Doctor's

COMMON SENSE HEALTH MANUAL

Parker Publishing Company, Inc.

West Nyack, N.Y.

Dedication

For those who, through illness of mind or body, have faltered, but not given up.

This book is a reference work based on research by the author. The opinions expressed herein are not necessarily those of or endorsed by the publisher. The directions stated in this book are in no way to be considered as a substitute for consultation with a duly licensed doctor.

Library of Congress Cataloging in Publication Data

Hurdle, J. Frank
   A country doctor's common sense health manual.

   1. Medicine, Popular. 2. Hygiene. I. Title.
[DNLM: 1. Hygience--Popular works. QT180 H962c]
RC81.H937   616   74-26873
ISBN 0-13-184358-3

Printed in the United States of America

What This Book Can Do For You

As a medical practitioner in rural and small town areas for many years, I've learned how to improve general health by showing patients like yourself how to prevent serious disease and how to deal with about 75 percent of ailments that send city people flocking to doctors' offices. This book is the essence of what I've helped thousands of people do to take care of their health. You might say this book is a manual of "country medicine"—a unique home treatment program that has worked near miracles for thousands of people.

You will find that the application of a few sound principles coupled with a generous helping of common sense will improve your general well-being, enable you to deal with most medical problems that may arise, and will aid you in staving off many of the ravages of chronic disease by preventing them from happening in the first place.

Some city practitioners seem bent on drugging patients to the point that it becomes necessary to maintain a drugstore in patients' homes! It also has started an entirely new medical problem—that of dealing with disease produced by all the drugs themselves!

How nice it would be if you could throw off the yoke of illness and begin feeling better without so many drugs. You can do just that by following the simple guidelines in this book and by applying to your own health problems the accounts of the many patients whose cases I describe.

In this book you'll find what I've learned in 23 years' experience practicing in small towns and in the country to be the most efficient and the most helpful methods and treatments for a wide variety of common illnesses and diseases.

For example, you'll find the best way to deal with being overweight (the cause of untold medical problems as you'll learn), and the best way to lick chronic fatigue or a painful gut that doesn't seem to function in the way you'd like. I say "best" because experience has taught me where I've been wrong in many instances in treating many conditions, and I'm afraid that experience is what makes most "experts" falter since they lack this essential ingredient.

7

All sorts of cults and schools of healing have arisen. It's impossible to absorb all of these approaches, but when you look closely, you find that they all have one thing in common. They depend for their success on confidence—confidence in the healer by the patient. This book will give you the confidence you need to help you with your health—it will give you confidence in *yourself*, the ultimate confidence needed by every person to remain physically and mentally well no matter what your particular approach to health may be.

First of all, I show you in this book how to revitalize your system—key up its reservoirs of resistance and defense so that you can ward off disease and infection. For those of you who have read one of my previous books, *Low Blood Sugar, a Doctor's Guide to Its Effective Control,* you now realize what an important part the smooth coordination of mind, body and spirit plays in the business of maintaining good health. You can reach this state of smooth concert of mind and body by following the advice in this book.

Furthermore, my experience in dealing with health problems in smaller communities and in rural areas has made it mandatory that patients learn for themselves how to cope with a variety of problems. This experience will be brought directly to you and you will be able to apply it immediately and easily to your own situation.

You can, by following my advice, change the entire character of your body and personality in six or eight short weeks so that even your friends and family will be amazed at the change. You'll become a happier, healthier more confident person, and, with the help of your own medical advisor, do wonders for your body and mind.

In answer to a perfectly reasonable skepticism you may have about what I've just said, consider the following: The human organism is a fantastic piece of biological machinery capable of feats that not even the most modern and up-to-date scientists yet realize. Not one in a million people have learned to utilize this marvelous system to its fullest capacity.

This book is designed to point the way for doing just that. To show you how you can reach the fullest potential of sound health. I don't propose that you will suddenly turn into a superman, but I do propose to you methods to bring to bear all the forces at your body's command to reach good health and to keep this enviable state for the rest of your life.

Start reading now to find extended limits to your health. Find how others have done it.

J. Frank Hurdle, M.D.

Contents

Benefits of Common Sense Health Control: *(The usual medical approach)* . *(A new approach)* . *(How Ruth got well)* . How to Get in Touch with Common Sense Health . How a Professor Learned Something New About Health: *(The professor triumphs)* . How Margie Made Secrets of Common Sense Health Work for Her: *(One important thing Margie learned)* . How Dave Discovered Better Health . Health Control Works for You Twenty-Four Hours a Day: *(How Susan found the benefits of common sense health)* . Health Control and Surgery . How Common Sense Health Control Pays Off for You . How Diabetes and High Blood Pressure Were Reversed Without Medicines: *(What Ellen was able to accomplish)* . Secrets of Health Control Revealed . Summary

Keeping Your Body Surging with Energy: *(How Lois T. gave up poor health)* . Physical Fitness—How It's Done: *(How Ben profited from his toning program)* . The Bonus of Physical Toning: *(Here's how you gain from your effort)* . How to Get Mind and Body Working Together for Your Health: *(How Mary O. won her full health)* . Further Bonuses of Physical Tone . How, When, and Where to Exercise. How a Doctor Works at Toning: *(The before bedtime routine)* . *(The tranquillizer routines)* . *(How to tone your face)* . *(What really happened in the doctor's routine)* . How Physical Toning Increases Resistance to Disease . Start Your Program Today for Extra Benefits: *(Hormones beefed up)* . *(New blood manufactured)* . *(Better antibodies produced)* . Looking, Feeling and Acting Younger Through Physical Toning: *(How Julia got big dividends of*

nerves) . How Low Blood Sugar Control Helps Your Nerves .
Your Program to Control Low Blood Sugar . A Guide to the Care
and Feeding of Your Brain: *(How to increase your awareness)* .
Lee Anne's Awareness Adventure: *(Awaken your brain)* . *(Enjoy
the same benefits Lee Anne found!)* . *(Look closely around you)* .
How to Prevent Alcohol from Dulling Your Brain: *(The beginning of
the end)* . *(Vitamin B can help you)* . How to Live with Your
Nerves . Summary

How to Prevent Urinary Infection: *(How flushing action helps your
kidneys and bladder)* . *(Follow this easy routine for flushing your
your kidney)* . *(How flushing works for you)* . Can You Strain
Your Kidneys?: *(How your physical toning brings on better elimina-
tion)* . *(How to protect your urine reservoir)* . How to Have Healthy
Kidneys: *(Good health principles makes better kidneys)* . *(A good
rule of thumb)* . How to Achieve Common Sense Acid-Base Balance
. How Alma Controlled Too Much Alkaline . Follow This Routine to
Maintain Acid-Alkaline Balance . How to Avoid Kidney Damaging
Infections . How to Start Your Kidney Protection Program Today .
Changing a Sluggish Bladder to a Healthy One . How Walt Overcame
Bladder Difficulties . How Cathy Overcame Bladder "Let-Down" .
Follow Cathy's Program for Healthy Bladder Tone: *(Here is a
special routine for females to help strengthen their bladder)* .
How to Avoid Kidney Stones: *(What happens with a hang-up)* .
You Can Profit from the Stone Prevention Program . A "Stone
Former" Achieves Good Health . How to Take Care of Your Prostate
(Inflammation—a trouble maker) . *(How massage helps)* . How You
Can Keep Your Prostate Working Smoothly. The Self-Help Prostatic
Massage Routine: *(Here is how you can recognize telltale signs of
prostate trouble)* . *(How to enjoy good health for your cervix and
uterus)* . *(Clarie's cervix problems and how she solved them)* . *(You can
reverse the stretching of childbirth)* . Menstruation and How You
Can Recognize Trouble with it . How to Handle Vaginal Infections :
(How to recognize yeast infection) . *(How to recognize trichomonas
infection)* . What to Do About Venereal Disease: *(Why VD is up)* .
(Playing it safe after contact) . *(The domino effect of VD)* . How
to Recognize VD in the Male . How to Recognize VD in the Female .
Summary

Moles and How to Tell a Bad One . How to Deal with Warts . Your Best Methods for Attractive Hair and Teeth: *(Caring for your hair)* . Using Clay's Program for Your Falling Hair . How Hilda Stopped Balding . How to Hang onto Your Teeth: *(Proper care of your teeth)* . *(Good dental care is a must)* . Summary

How to Relieve Stiff, Aching Muscles: *(How to control muscle spasms)* . Your Stiff Muscle Routine: *(How to overcome strains and sprains)* . Your Five Point Sprain Management Program . How to Master Strapping Techniques: *(How to strap an ankle)* . *(How to strap a knee)* . *(How to strap an injured chest)* . *(How to strap a back)* . How to Maintain a Healthy Back: *(How to combat house-wives' back)* . Your Program for a Healthy Back: *(What to do with serious back injuries)* . How These People Overcame Common Injuries . How to Handle Arthritis: *(Dealing with rheumatoid arthritis)* Your Guide for Rheumatoid Arthritis Control . How Carol Controlled Stress, for Control of Rheumatoid Arthritis: *(How to deal with osteoarthritis)* . *(How to deal with gouty arthritis)* . The Proper Care of Your Feet . Summary

How to Deal with Headaches: *(Nerves and blood vessels can be troublemakers)* . How to Detect Migraine Headaches . How June Battled Her Migraines: *(June's program can help you with migraine)* . *(Migraine's bark is much worse than its bite)* . How to Ease Sinus Problems: *(How to watch for sinus problems)* . *(More sinus aids than people)* . Your Sinus Treatment Guide . Al's Success with Sinus Can Also Be Yours . How to Handle Ear Problems: *(How ear, sinus, and nose all interact with each other)* . How to Keep Your Ears Healthy . Let Ken's Experience Help Your Ears: *(Ear opening hints for your use)* . *(How to take care of your eardrums)* . *(How to rid yourself of unwanted wax)* . *(Keeping solid objects out of your ear canals)* . How to Cope with Eye Problems: *(How to handle "red eye")* . *(What to do about eye muscle problems)* . How Karen Regained Her Vision: *(How to tell when your vision needs attention)* . *(What you can do with eye injuries)* . Your Guide to Cinder Removal: *(Putting the injured eye at rest)* . *(Don't make Laura's mistake)* . What You Can Do About Nose Problems . The Critical Questions to Ask About Nose Injuries: *(Handling long nasal hairs)* . *(Nosebleeds)* . How to Stop Most Nosebleeds . How Mel's Nosebleed Was Stopped . Summary

1

How to Make Secrets of Common Sense Health Work for You

The more I see people with health problems, the more it's necessary to get across the idea of health control for true healing. Health control is simply this—doing all you can to *prevent* trouble before it starts. It's getting your system in shape so that you've done everything you can to stop serious problems before they start.

There's good reason for this preventive outlook. It's estimated that 80 percent of the major illnesses suffered by people today can be prevented! A good reason, I think, for looking at health as something which you can help first of all by looking at your body. Looking at it with these ideas in mind: What can I do to improve my health control? What is there that needs to be brought in line? And how can I do it?

I'd like to examine the answers to this question and show you how you can bring your health into line by following my "country doctor" programs that others have found work for them quickly and satisfactorily.

BENEFITS OF COMMON SENSE HEALTH CONTROL

One of the most miserable persons I've ever known was Ruth R., a lady who lived on a farm near the town where I practiced. Ruth stands out in my mind because in trying to help this poor lady get over a host of ailments, the idea of health control hit me like a sledge hammer. Since then, I've used health control successfully with many hundreds of patients.

Ruth was at the bottom of her health ladder—she was 70

pounds overweight; had gall bladder trouble; had severe varicose veins of both legs, and swelling of her ankles. She had sore, stiff, and enlarged joints and, as a matter of fact, there wasn't an organ in her body that didn't have trouble. Ruth was not an old person—only 37—but she had deteriorated in health until she looked, acted, and felt like 73!

The Usual Medical Approach

As was my habit in those earlier days, and as is the habit of far too many practitioners today, I started to treat each of her separate complaints. Soon she was on pills to reduce, pills for gallbladder trouble, pills for her ankle swelling, pills for her sore joints. Does all this sound familiar? I had to sharply curtail her activities because of the varicose veins in her legs.

A New Approach

Then I began to mull over Ruth's problem. Ruth was far too young, far too bright a person to shackle with all this medicine and inactivity. She certainly couldn't get the rest she needed being a farmer's wife—you can't run a farm or anything else if you're confined to your backside all day. There must be a better way, I thought. Surely, Ruth hadn't always been in this fix. What had happened?

Carefully, painstakingly, Ruth and I talked about the past—how she used to feel; what changed; why she overate; her health habits. I discovered that Ruth had lapsed into a lethargy where body, mind and spirit had disintegrated and drifted, each to a dark corner of its own—each lost to the old spark of vitality and vigor necessary for healthful living.

Slowly, Ruth and I managed to rediscover the real Ruth. We both began to see that what we were doing in treating all the symptoms of her many diseases was a poor approach. Poor because we had not reached the basic problem—had not come to grips with the causes of all her ailments. We had not gotten *inside* Ruth to work from there to the outside, but rather we had only scratched the surface, and they were weak scratches at that.

How Ruth Got Well

The first thing Ruth and I did together was to look at health control. The real Ruth was exposed—what she saw there and what she thought she'd want things to be like. What we both saw was chaos.

We started with Ruth's weight problem. She was unhappy with her life on the farm and was basically a lonely woman. We got her husband in on the act. We got Ruth's mind focused on prevention. She was able to stick to a reducing diet for the first time in years after numerous failures. Why? Because now she had something to hang on to—the real Ruth was guiding her efforts. She used her willpower to control her appetite and to make herself stick to dieting. Between diet and exercise she lost 35 pounds in three months! I'll show you how Ruth did this at home in Chapter 2.

With weight and diet control came an abrupt end to Ruth's constant gassiness, indigestion, and abdominal pain—the chief signs of gallbladder upset. With her nagging gallbladder trouble out of the way, Ruth perked up mentally even more. And as her weight fell even further toward normal, so did the nagging joint pains and ankle swelling. At this point, Ruth was able to throw away three of her medicines. With the drugs out of Ruth's system, she was able to really get down to business with health control—she stayed with weight reduction until she'd lost the 70 pounds excess and then dropped eight more pounds in addition! She never felt better in her life!

Ruth saved herself not only a life of crippling joint destruction, heart disease and gallstones, but she also came to know herself better *from the inside out.* She corrected the lonely aspect of her life by starting a family (something she'd been unable to do before) and began organizing friends and neighbors into a health unit for the purpose of bringing better health practices into their community.

Today Ruth is very active in her rural community projects. She's happy because she spends a lot of time helping others, and she has plenty of reserve energy to do everything she needs to do as a housewife on a farm. And she hasn't had a sick day in ten years!

HOW TO GET IN TOUCH WITH COMMON SENSE HEALTH

To size up your health—to stand next to it and have a good look—you need to know its parts. These parts are the systems of your body. These systems are the parts that control the very essence of your health, and when they're working *together as a unit*—in complete harmony, one complementing the other in balanced proportion—continuing health and happiness in daily living can be yours.

What makes things work as they do in your body? What outside effects change the progress of your health? They are numerous, but they are easy to control and use for good health. All these benefits are yours in following the guidelines in this book.

HOW A PROFESSOR LEARNED SOMETHING NEW ABOUT HEALTH

A middle-aged professor of agronomy who taught at the agricultural college in the small town I practiced in had suffered from migraine headaches for years—since he was 18 years old, as a matter of fact. Dr. Will A. had been given the usual bank of medicines—some to prevent migraine headaches; others to take when he actually got an attack. His headaches were getting to be quite incapacitating—they'd knock him out sometimes for two or three days. In addition, Will was one of those people who seemed to have one cold after another. Some would end up in his chest, others were secondary infections, and still others would cause bronchitis, and even pneumonia on occasion. His colds seemed to get more frequent and severe in direct proportion to his migraine headaches.

Will was assigned a tour of duty to India as a visiting agricultural expert. The thought of being so far away from his home, his doctors and his medicines actually brought on another migraine attack the day he learned of his assignment.

Taking a clue from Ruth's spectacular performance, I had a long talk with Will shortly before he was to leave. The topic of our conversation—Will's health control.

I pointed out to Will the startling relationship between his colds, bronchitis attacks and his migraine headaches. We began to talk about Will's system, what makes it tick; his expectations; his frustrations; his joys and griefs. He began to take a look at himself—the very foundation upon which the individual called Professor Will was built. He saw himself as having become a man *controlled by*, instead of *in control* of his surroundings.

The Professor Triumphs

Will learned what things caused his migraine attacks. He began to realize that it was an overanxious desire to perform at far beyond his own abilities—to attempt to do things on his own that ordinarily three people should be doing; to settle for no less than absolute perfection in everything; and other tension producing habits.

I showed Will that the physical cause of his migraine headaches was a two-stage reaction to all this *overdoing it* kind of thing. First, the blood vessels inside his skull overreacted by clamping down so that their inside bore was reduced to a fraction of their usual diameter. This effect produces the *aura* that people suffering from migraine often have—peculiar vision difficulties like flashing lights or dark spots running about their visual fields, dizzy sensations and many others. Shortly after this clamping down, the blood vessels suddenly relax and just the opposite takes place: they dilate and expand. This sudden expansion stretches the walls of the blood vessels producing the typical *vascular headache* of migraine—the one-side-of-the-skull excruciating pain often accompanied by nausea and vomiting.

By understanding that this blood vessel reaction caused his migraine, Will was able, in an amazingly short time, to actually stop the second phase of his migraine—the incapacitating headaches. He did this by concentrating on his blood vessels when phase one appeared—by preventing the blood vessels inside his head from expanding and then returning to normal size. It worked a charm. You'll be able to learn Will's method at home. It's found in Chapter 3.

When the professor returned from his stint in India, I talked to him about his health and he told me that he'd been able to reduce the number of his migraines by half! This he did by altering his way of life. He eliminated the perfectionism and learned to delegate responsibility to others. He didn't allow life to overwhelm him. In other words, Will was approaching health control. I have no doubt whatsoever that eventually his migraine headaches will be completely eliminated.

An interesting postscript to Will's case is that since returning from India he hasn't had a single cold or the flu and that's been a record for nine years now!

HOW MARGIE MADE SECRETS OF COMMON SENSE HEALTH WORK FOR HER

Another good example of health control is seen in a patient of mine named Margie S. Margie was in her early twenties when I first saw her with a weight problem. She'd been through all the usual fad diets and had taken virtually all the weight pills known at the time. All this effort was to no avail. She'd lose a little weight for a short period of time, but would soon have it all back again and more.

What was Margie missing? She was, for one thing, trying to lose weight without starting a regular exercise routine at the same time. She was trying to knock off weight (to force herself to stay on diets) leaving her physical body to drift about on its own.

When Margie first came to me, I told her I'd help her if she'd promise to follow instructions and stop taking all sorts of drugs to curb her appetite. She was very surprised when she realized that the pills she'd taken weren't *to make her lose weight* as many people like Margie insist they do, but rather to artificially knock down her appetite. When she accepted this, Margie was ready for the next step: To start a reducing diet *and an exercise routine at the same time.*

One Important Thing Margie Learned

It was touch and go at first, but I kept reminding her about her promise. Margie learned several things within the first three weeks. The most important thing she learned was that her exercise routine *made her diet a lot easier to stick to.* In fact, she was able to take in *fewer* calories than was actually called for in her restricted diet—and at *no extra effort to her willpower, and without drugs.* Why was this? Simple. Every time Margie went through her exercise routine, a chain of events occurred as follows:

1. Toning of muscle cells increased the elimination of waste products that always accumulate in lazy, unused muscle cells.
2. Forcing millions of muscle cells to work for the first time in years began to increase the power of each cell which in turn toned up the small nerve endings in and around these cells.
3. The refreshed nerve cells speeded up transmission between brain and muscles, increasing tone of brain cells controlling newly exercised muscles.
4. Renewed vigor of brain cells increased Margie's capacity to *stick to* her diet and exercise.

Margie discovered one of the great bonuses of working with health control: Starting with her physical well-being helped her mental well-being and the new, stronger combination of the two spurred her onward with the spirit to continue to the end of the goal, namely, to lose weight and to permanently keep it within normal range.

With this relatively simple act of health control, Margie, who is now socially popular and in demand by male friends, gained control of her body. In doing so, she insured that her various systems would never be ravaged by such disease states as diabetes, cardiac and blood vessel trouble, high blood pressure, arthritis, and a host of ailments that would fill a medical book.

Today, Margie is happily married and the mother of three healthy children all of whom, you can rest assured, are learning about common sense health at an early age.

HOW DAVE DISCOVERED BETTER HEALTH

Dave B. is an example of a man burning the candle at both ends, making a lot of money while doing so, but slowly killing his health in the process. Dave was a gentleman farmer, a bank director and a cattle-ranch operator. A usual day consisted of steady waves of crises, one piling on top of another. He'd already acquired an ulcer and had given up about 50 percent of his stomach to the surgeon. When the remaining stomach wasn't upset, his bowel was cramping or he had either diarrhea or severe constipation. He was miserable. His family was miserable. But his bank account was fat.

When I first saw Dave, he was just a year past his stomach surgery and was well on his way toward another ulcer at the spot where they'd sewn his stomach to his intestine. He was taking drugs to keep him awake at night so he could stay up to date on his business interests and these were followed by sedatives to make him sleep. And he was on three kinds of medicine for bowel trouble. I asked him after the first couple of visits if he'd be interested in getting hold of his bowel problems without any drugs. He laughed nervously and suggested I must be "putting him on."

I introduced Dave to common sense health control. When we began to explore it, we found that it was simple conditioning at the source of Dave's health problems. He finally accepted the fact that his gut was being used as a *sounding board* for all his frustrations, setbacks, excess nervous energy and anger. Literally everything that upset Dave or went against his grain was routed through the two large nerves that control the stomach and intestine. Dave was beating his gut to a pulp without realizing it.

The first thing Dave had to learn was the nature of this rerouting of nervous energy. He had to understand what was going on and finally mold the solution for it—the addition of a safety valve to blow off steam and excess nervous energy built up from the pressures and strains of the day. And he had to learn to do this *before* it was delivered by his nervous system into his gut.

Dave learned this rather quickly. During a period of about three months, Dave spent enough time with his health program to begin to shape his health differently. He learned to vent anger and frustration through properly suited channels of physical exertion and blowing his stack—usually in one of his cattle feeding lots where only the Hereford cows could hear him.

He practiced the art of concentration on the muscles that control his bowel—the ones that contract and knot up to cause cramps. He learned to sense when the cramps were coming on and was able to stop them in their tracks merely by making his gut relax. He was able to stop the cramps, the diarrhea and the constipation. No more anti-cramp drugs, no more laxatives and no more pain! All this was accomplished through health control as given in this book.

HEALTH CONTROL WORKS FOR YOU
TWENTY-FOUR HOURS A DAY

There is no limit to the uses of health control. I know several people who even use it to solve problems. All you have to do to utilize this rather striking bonus of health control is to suggest to yourself, just before you're ready to doze off to sleep at night, that you will awaken with the solution to whatever problem is on your mind. Then forcefully put any and all thoughts about the problem completely from your conscious thinking and have a relaxing and restful sleep.

The next day—sometimes even later that night—you will have the solution popping right into your mind from nowhere. Sometimes it awakens you at three o'clock in the morning, the answer to the seemingly insolvable problem shining in your mind like a neon sign. This is why a number of people I know keep a pencil and a pad of notepaper on their nightstands or dressers. When they wake up with such answers pushing their way out, they jot down every detail on paper so that they won't forget it in the morning.

Once you've attained health control, it does indeed go right on working for you even when you're asleep!

There is no age limit for health control. Neither is there a limit to what it may accomplish, given persistence, practice and a little imagination.

How Susan Found the Benefits of Common Sense Health

A young mother-to-be, Susan C. exemplifies this diversity. Susan was expecting in about a month, and suddenly she began to sob and wail in my office one day. It was her first baby, and she was understandably nervous. When she finally calmed down, she admitted a dread fear of her upcoming delivery. It seems that her grandmother had a terrible time with pain; her mother had a similarly terrible time with pain delivering Susan, and Susan was positive she was destined for the same fate.

Susan and I explored the possibilities of common sense health. (Nowadays, it's called natural childbirth.) When her delivery time came, she called me on the phone and I suggested to her, through prearranged conditioning, that she should relax completely and have no more pain with her labor contractions.

Susan had no more arrived at the hospital than she delivered a bouncing baby boy. Her first, second, and third stages of labor had lasted no more than about an hour and a half and she required no anesthesia whatsoever.

HEALTH CONTROL AND SURGERY

Another patient of mine, Paul F., age 39, mastered things so well that he was able to be up and walking, his back straight as an arrow and feeling absolutely no distress, within 30 minutes after an operation to correct a large hernia.

Hundreds of patients have learned to master health control for better physical efficiency. I know of not a single one who has taken time to do so who didn't say, "Why didn't someone tell me about this before?" or "When I think of all the time and money I've wasted and all the misery I've suffered . . . it's unbelievable!"

HOW COMMON SENSE HEALTH CONTROL PAYS OFF FOR YOU

You may still be asking yourself, will it pay to try for health control? Is it worth the effort? How will my health actually benefit from it? These are legitimate questions.

What it means, what reaching toward health control and making it work for your total well-being means is that *regardless of your present state of health and regardless of what you've had to go through with illness and infirmities that afflict the human organism,* you can achieve lasting, permanent health! If this is not a good reason for "bothering" I'm afraid I don't understand what a good reason is.

In other words, doesn't it seem logical that the first step toward the goal of lasting health would be in the field of preventing as much disease as you possibly can *before* it starts?

You can take advantage of this preventive method today regardless of what state your health may be in at this time. You can begin to head off trouble that may already have started, and you can begin your journey down the road to permanent and glorious good health now by taking advantage of what follows in this book. And you needn't blame yourself for not having started sooner—*it's never too late to master health control!*

HOW DIABETES AND HIGH BLOOD PRESSURE WERE REVERSED WITHOUT MEDICINES

When I first met Ellen J., a lady in her mid fifties and heading for an early grave because of poor health, she was resigned to a life—a short one at that—of chronic illness and continuous treatment with enough medicines to fill a doctor's bag. She was convinced she was born to suffer, and there was the question whether she might already have come to depend on prolonged poor health for psychological well-being!

She had had diabetes for about five years. She also had begun to develop hypertension—high blood pressure—severe enough to require drugs to bring it under control. This combination of two major diseases can kill quickly, even in young people. Her chance of having a stroke within two or three years was about six in ten; of having a blood vessel problem severe enough to close off blood supply in an arm, leg or vital organ about seven in ten.

You wouldn't think it possible that people in their right mind would hesitate to do anything at all if they could have prevented arriving at such a state. Yet over the years, I've seen thousands of people doing just that! Putting themselves in the completely unrealistic position of suffering, disease, and crippling because they didn't know or perhaps didn't care that what they were doing might prove fatal.

What Ellen Was Able to Accomplish

Ellen was now in a position to listen to reason since her disease states had progressed to the point of virtual incapacitation at a time in life when she had much to do, much to live for, and a family which depended on her.

By reaching for health control, Ellen was able to accomplish the following change in an almost unbelievable fashion:

1. Through proper dieting and exercise, she lost 60 pounds of excess flab and was able to tone up muscles to the extent of controlling her diabetes with only two oral tablets of medicine a day instead of the 45 units of insulin she had used before.
2. Within three months after accomplishing step one, Ellen's blood pressure returned to normal levels—*without medicines of any kind!*
3. Within a year of accomplishing steps one and two, Ellen halted the recurrent infections, blood vessel damage and nerve destruction that diabetes causes.
4. Five years later, Ellen has remained the picture of dynamic health; has become active in community affairs; has become once again the wifely companion to her husband of bygone years and has the energy and zip of a person 20 years her junior.

And I can assure you that Ellen added about 20 sparkling years of healthful life by her accomplishments. Moreover, she has assured herself that neither heart attack nor stroke will be a part of her life; she has removed herself from the doomed-to-suffer list of hundreds of thousands of people who have not been fortunate enough to learn and practice health control.

If I can show you in this book how to practice the art of health control, you too will benefit as the patients whose actual case histories I've used in this chapter have benefitted. And if you're fortunate enough to have preserved your body from some of the infirmities these patients have suffered, your benefits will be all the more striking!

SECRETS OF HEALTH CONTROL REVEALED

The point to be remembered is this: You have in your body the ingredients necessary to heal ills; to prevent their occurrences as well as their reoccurrences and to lift yourself up to greater heights of physical and mental accomplishments. I am going to show you how to do it. How to harness your body systems for efficient, healthful use. How to start down the road to health control using what you've got inside you as the foundation to building a better heart, lungs, blood vessels, internal organs, nerves, bones, muscles and skin. Once you've acquired this key in maintaining excellent health, using the methods and treatments I'll give you for dealing with ailments that come along to all of us, you should be able to count vigorous healthful years and mental achievement beyond your dreams among your most valuable possessions.

SUMMARY

1. Your body systems are the essence of health regardless of present or past states of health. You can learn how to control them easily and how to care for them when they go on the blink.
2. Prevention is and always has been desired over waiting for something to happen and then trying to deal with it. You can prevent 80 percent of the ailments that befall mankind today by reaching for health control.
3. Health control is the basis for all the past health cults down through the ages and remains the basis for modern medical science even though it has taken second place to treatments and cures in this age of the miracle drug.
4. This book is to point the way to your health control and to show you how to deal with the various ailments that befall most of us, and how to overcome them.
5. Here, in short, are tried-and-true techniques of "Country Medicine" that you can use to cure or relieve a wide variety of ailments right in the privacy of your own home. With this help, you should keep strong and well—and live to a ripe old age.

2

How to Build Resistance to Diseases, Reverse Low Blood Sugar and Halt the Aging Process

This chapter will show you how you can surge vigorous, fresh, new energy through your body. How, at any age, you can begin to build your body into an impregnable fortress, resistant to disease, rack and wear. In short, how physical fitness works to toughen your health.

To begin with you can start today with your physical toning routine. This section will show you how to do just that. You'll see the difference; you'll feel the difference. You'll be well on your way to amazing health after you've mastered this material.

Besides building resistance to virtually all the maladies that wear down your health, you'll begin to look, feel and act younger after only a few weeks on the routines. Recall the cases in the first chapter? Well, now *you* get *your* chance. It's your turn to stop, walk away from the rat race just long enough to find out how, when, and where to start feeling like a human being again.

There will also be a discussion about diet in this section. You'll see how this business of diet can be handled without drugs, gimmicks or fancy menus.

KEEPING YOUR BODY SURGING WITH ENERGY

Right there—locked in your own body—is the first key to lasting health! The secret of the ages? long-hidden mysteries of some forgotten cult? Buried mysteries of ancient Egyptians? No! *Physical toning is the answer.*

"How could this be?" you ask. "Is this the secret sought after by thousands through the ages?" Yes, indeed. Listen to Lois T.'s story to see exactly what I mean.

How Lois T. Gave Up Poor Health

Case in Point: Lois T., age 30, single, thin, frail and fragile. A do-nothing who hardly ever moved a muscle, and complained of the pain if she did do so!

Complaint: Lack of interest in anything; forced to bed with the simplest cold, of which she had at least two every month; nervous, dizzy and fainted at the merest change of surroundings; upset stomach; nervous bladder, forever getting infected, thus necessitating antibiotics.

Physical Activity: Practically none—just a minimum to *get around.*

Condition of Health Control: Really terrible!

Prognosis: Very poor indeed if continued. Will never taste life or appreciate what living is all about. Will develop numerous chronic ailments (mostly imagined) and become medicine dependent (medicines for every symptom). Even so, this condition Lois had was completely reversible!

Diagnosis: Poor energy turnover; low blood sugar; disintegrated health control with poor resistance and out-of-balance nervous system.

Prescription: Exercise routines twice a day—first thing in the morning, and last thing before bedtime. Stop all medicines.

Result: Lois felt the surge of energy through tired, worn, toneless muscles for the first time since reaching adulthood. It wasn't easy for her—she ached in every bone of her body even though she started on her toning routines with the simplest of exercises and for only two or three minutes at a time. Gradually, however, in about three weeks there was a change. Lois admitted she felt better, ate better, and had in general a brighter outlook on what had previously been a dull life.

Her low blood sugar levels came up to normal, and through proper dieting Lois was able to keep it steady throughout the day. After this milestone, she found she was able to increase the strenuousness of her exercises and gradually worked her way up to 20 and 30 minutes twice a day. She gained weight—where it counted most, and in firm, well-toned muscle tissue—not flab and fat. As this change developed, Lois' popularity increased and she became a delightful companion for both men and women friends.

Both the frequent colds and the nervous bladder symptoms gradually disappeared and since then, Lois hasn't had a *poor day* in years! Lois found out that there is, indeed, something to health control, and she now enjoys physical well-being as a result of her efforts.

PHYSICAL FITNESS—HOW IT'S DONE

Just make up your mind today that fitness is going to become as much a part of your everyday life as mealtime and brushing your teeth. That you're at least willing to give it a try. If you do, I'll guarantee that after six short weeks, *you won't want to stop because you'll feel so much better!*

I had a real "go-around" about this very point with a man named Ben J. Ben was 28, father of two boys, farmed three sections of land with his father and brothers and was well on his way to trouble at his early age. Why? His blood pressure was 40 points above normal for someone of Ben's age! And this is exactly what causes our old friend, the stroke.

Of course, when you looked at Ben, it was obvious that something was wrong: He was about 80 pounds overweight! And his back kept "going out" on him.

How Ben Profited from His Toning Program

"Exercise? Me? I'm as strong as an ox!" said Ben. And he was at least partially right. He could heft a hundred pound sack of feed with either arm—but his belly sagged (stretched-out abdominal muscles), and his "bad back" indicated weakness of back muscles as well.

It's going to be your job," I replied to Ben's comment, "to make your belly and your back as strong as your arms are. And with an added bonus—to get your blood pressure down before it blows a gasket!" Ben got serious. He decided to do what I advised. Here's what happened:

Twice a day, Ben worked on his back muscles. First thing he did at five in the morning when he arose (before chores) was to do cradle rocks and ten sit-ups. Ben swore at me at our next meeting—he found out his ox-like strength was confined to his arms and chest—because the routines really racked him up for six weeks. Finally it stopped hurting so much—he increased the number of cradle rocks and added double bends to his routine, then added some thigh and side muscle exercises for ten more minutes before bedtime (except on week-ends when I let him off the hook).

He put a bed board in his bed; learned how to lift heavy objects *correctly* and mastered back pack techniques (all these techniques discussed in detail later). Ben also cut 1500 carbohydrate calories from his diet and replaced them with protein calories.

In six months, Ben lost 45 pounds and by the end of the year, he shed the remaining excess of 35 pounds. His blood pressure returned to normal, however, after only two and a half months—a tribute to how well the human organism can function if given only half a chance! And I never did put Ben on any medicines.

Miracle? Coincidence? Lucky? Well, maybe so, but the fact is Ben just grabbed hold of health control with those strong arms of his and shaped it up. He utilized what he had going for him to restore his health—possibly preventing a lifetime of crippling health from stroke and a permanently lame back. All I know is that Ben is now a model of good health—he keeps his back in shape with far less toning than it took to restore health to it; his blood pressure has remained normal, and will continue to do so unless he gains back the weight; and Ben found out that toning increased his capacity to keep up with heavy farm work by 50 percent.

THE BONUS OF PHYSICAL TONING

Look at it this way—you are perhaps one of those people who has tried toning in the past without much success. You gave up because it was too hard or you couldn't break the habit of sitting on your tail when you were done with your day's work, or you were in too big a hurry when you got up in the morning. Try one more time, following any one of hundreds of variations in the routines I'll talk about in a minute *and you will also strengthen your willpower and your mental capacity at the same time!*

Here's How You Gain from Your Effort

1. Consider the *magic circle* to be muscle—glands—nerves—glands—brain. The five points are tightly bound together and remember, surging power can go *both ways.*

2. You start at the muscle point on the circle. Power is generated in muscle cells; travels to one or more glands; travels to nerves; travels to brain.

3. Brain cells (including those controlling your mind) are energized. Surge of energy back through glands; to nerves; to other glands or directly back to muscle cells.

4. Constant daily stimulation of brain from muscles increases brain cells' efficiency and sharpness. Mental capacity advances to new heights.

5. Soon, magic circle is bulging with two-way energy bursts. And all because of the fact that you've decided to start your circle humming with renewed activity by starting daily fitness routines! Mind and muscle working together—one increasing the efficiency of the other.

Yes, it's fantastic. The human organism is one of the most

fantastic packages of equipment in the world. You have the ability—right there in *your* organism as it exists today—to start changes that may completely alter your future health and well-being. To ward off 75 percent of the blights to your health and utilize simple techniques to easily overcome the remaining 25 percent! Why not start this evening or tomorrow morning at the latest? It will be the best time investment you ever made.

HOW TO GET MIND AND BODY WORKING TOGETHER FOR YOUR HEALTH

There is no end to the ways in which health control works for your well-being. I recall Mary O's case because it's directly to the point and simple.

How Mary O. Won Her Full Health

Mary was a thin, 40 year old, small town "single lady" when I first met her. She was highly nervous and had high blood pressure. She was a chain smoker and used alcohol moderately, though for Mary, moderately was far too much.

After only a three months' twice-daily physical toning routine and having cut both cigarettes and alcohol by 75 percent and learning how to make natural health work for her, Mary quickly got rid of high blood pressure. She lost her *nervous Nellie* personality; gained 25 pounds of solid weight spread evenly over arms, legs, breasts, and thighs and was married within a year! All this even though she was afraid of men before—a frail neurotic headed for health problems and a life of both real and imaginary sickness. And all it took was 15 or 20 minutes twice a day to bring about these changes!

In Mary's case, her vastly improved health extended right down into her subconscious mind to bring about *personality* changes that literally made a new woman out of her. Control of Mary's physical tone helped her out as well with her *emotions,* enabling her to become stable, strong and every inch a woman.

FURTHER BONUSES OF PHYSICAL TONE

No matter where you start with physical tone routines, you can't go wrong! Consider what happens when you do, say, 10 or 15 sit-ups in the evening:

1. Exertion of abdominal muscles forces deeper breathing.
2. Exertion of abdominal muscles forces faster heart action.
3. Exertion of abdominal muscles increases tone of blood vessels as blood surges through vessels faster and with more vigor.
4. Exertion of abdominal muscles compresses bowels to help eliminate constipation.

Think of it! By merely picking one set of muscles to tone at first, you've automatically also toned up lungs, heart, blood vessels and your intestinal tract! And the more toning you do, the more strength you add to lungs, heart and blood vessels. In the previous case, Mary added enough tone to her blood vessels to stop high blood pressure! You can do this and much more with toning routines.

As if this weren't *miracle* enough, there is more to come! Consider this series of events when you start your toning routines:

1. Recall the *magic circle* and how you tone up abdominal muscles by doing sit-ups.
2. Power surges from muscle cells to adrenal glands. Adrenal glands pour out adrenalin and vital hormones.
3. Adrenalin and hormones go to every gland in your body to stimulate their cells to pour out other hormones and actually make your muscle cells stronger and more responsive to the tone you're producing by contracting your stomach muscles.
4. Some of the hormones go to your brain where master hormones are released that stimulate appetite, settle down your intestinal tract, release emotional tension built up during the day, raise blood sugar, and stimulate your metabolism.
5. Creative thought processes to get what you want are released into your mind!

HOW, WHEN, AND WHERE TO EXERCISE

All the toning you need can be done in and around your house without any apparatus or special gimmicks whatsoever. The cardinal rules for toning are as follows:

1. Start out easy. Don't overtax at first; let the increases in numbers of movements done with your muscles come slowly but steadily.
2. If you're overweight (consult height-weight-frame tables at the end of the book) *start your reducing diet the first day you start toning up. There is no toning without diet; no dieting without toning.* If you're underweight, don't worry. Your toning will bring it up naturally.

3. Plan your toning routines to include *all* the muscles in your body, not just the larger ones, which are easily seen. The bigger your belly, the slower you must go, but the more important it is to start!

4. If you have ill health from whatever reason, this is *not* an excuse to skip toning—it simply means you must build your toning *around* the illness until you've gotten the illness under control.

5. Exercise *before* meals on an empty stomach! Exercise at least once during the day when you're at your best (first thing on getting up in the morning, for example) and once when you're through with your day (last thing before going to bed, for example).

A physician friend of mine uses the following toning routine to tremendous advantage. You can take hints from it, modify it to suit your particular needs, change it completely if you desire and most certainly introduce variations of your own. But do *your* toning routine at least twice a day. Start now!

HOW A DOCTOR WORKS AT TONING

Doctor Franklin, age 44 and married with four children, arises about seven in the morning. The first thing he does is to empty his bladder—sounds like this might go without saying, but it's important as you will note when you start. Next, Doctor Franklin works on his arms, shoulders and chest with various combinations of the following:

1. Pulls arms outwardly with fingers of both hands linked together securely; then pushes arms inwardly with the palms of both hands flattened against one another. Does this with fingertips or palms pressed together in front, waist high, and again in back behind neck; and in back waist high. This is to use several different muscle groups, though basically the same "push-pull" technique is used.

2. Pulls right forearm from straight out position to full flexion (pulls lower arm toward shoulder) while force is being applied by left hand to right hand—using one arm, in other words, to force outwardly as the other arm pulls inwardly. Then he reverses arms.

3. Pulls down with left hand on top of right shoulder while forcing upwardly with right shoulder. Reverses arms and shoulders.

4. Locks right hand around left elbow; left hand around right elbow (alternating front and back) waist high and pulls inwardly with both arms and hands—chest and upper back muscles toned in this manner.

5. Sucks in belly muscles after deep inspiration (breathing in) until abdomen quivers from strain; then breathes out (expires) and tightens up belly muscles by pulling them in downward direction.

6. Grabs right ankle with right hand, leg bent at the knee, and forces down with lower leg, arching back at same time. Then reverses hands and legs (one of the "cradle" toners that Ben J. used earlier).

Doctor Franklin then switches his attention to legs and lungs as follows:

1. Squats, legs fully bent at knees, arms straight out in front, then rises to standing position using only leg muscles, repeating rapidly 30 to 50 times.

2. Jogs in place. Lifts one thigh fully as high as possible, bending knee at same time; then the same with the other leg. Done rapidly, this is just like running down the street, or jogging, except there is no forward motion. He does this for five to seven minutes—the equivalent of about half to three-quarters of a mile of jogging. During summer months, Doctor Franklin actually jogs along the street, through a park or around the block as a substitute.

3. Stretches out on the floor, back straight, supported by his extended arms. Draws one leg up under him (like jogging in a horizontal position), then the reverse. Does this rapidly for three to five minutes.

4. Does straddle hops; standing straight, hands by sides, feet together, then suddenly spreading legs to the sides and extending arms over the head to touch hands; then back to the straight position again rapidly. For five or six minutes.

This ends the Doctor's morning routine, having toned up at least three quarters of his entire array of muscles in ten or fifteen minutes. In the evening, just before retiring, Doctor Franklin concentrates on "floor exercises" as follows:

The Before Bedtime Routine

1. Flat on floor on back; hands clasped behind neck; legs held straight and flat on floor. Does sit-ups—makes belly muscles pull him up to sitting position touching left elbow to right knee, then back down flat again, then sits up again, touching right elbow to left knee. Does 30 to 45 in rapid fire order.

2. Does scissor clamps; at the same time doing scissor kicks with legs, does sit-ups. Scissor kicks consist of elevating both legs about 12 to 18 inches off floor, laying flat on back; knees straight at all times; then swing both legs out to the sides as far as possible then swing both legs in, crossing right lower leg over left the first time, left leg crossed over right the second time. No touching the floor with heels or legs at any time.

3. Does push-ups. While stretched out, belly down toward the floor and supported by extended arms and balls of both feet (knees straight at all times), letting his arms drop him to almost touching the floor with his chin, then making arms raise him back up again to starting position. No knee or belly sagging during maneuvers! Repeats rapidly 30 to 50 times.

He then does either the *sleeper* or the *clown* routine.

The Tranquillizer Routines

Sleeper Routine: Standing straight, chin lowered to chest, hands clasped behind head, he forces his neck backward against the pressure of his clasped hands. When neck is fully bent back, he reverses his hands, holds them against his forehead and bends his head and neck forward against the pressure of his hands. Repeats this several times. Then right hand held against the side (temple area) of his head while head bent to left side (toward left shoulder), then forcing head and neck to bend to right against pressure of right hand. Then the opposite movement (head and neck forced to left against pressure of left hand at temple area). This with various positions of neck flexion and extension—in other words, head forced from side to side with the neck fully bent (chin on chest); partially bent (chin up a bit); then all the way back so that chin points to ceiling. Then a full rolling motion of the head and neck (like drawing an imaginary circle with nose), first in a clockwise direction, then counterclockwise. This maneuver is better for sleep than any tranquillizer known to medicine.

Doctor Franklin doesn't do *each* of these exercises *every* morning and night—he picks one or two from each category and concentrates on them on Monday, then mixes them around, one or two at a time, Tuesday through Friday. He gives himself a rest from Friday night to Sunday night, at which time he resumes his routines. He tells me he figures the yard work, house repairs and so on during the weekends and (in summer) getting out fishing and hiking and so on makes up for the lack of routines over the weekends.

How to Tone Your Face

He explains that the *clown routine* is his way of face muscle toning. He says you just relax (use a mirror if you want) and put your neck, chin, mouth, nose, cheek, eye and forehead muscles through every possible movement they are capable of making—straining them to the utmost with each grimace. "If my kids are watching me, and they laugh when they see me doing the *clown* toners, then I know I'm doing it right," Doctor Franklin says.

What Really Happened in the Doctor's Routine

Let's look at what Doctor Franklin's routines do for him. Notice first that he's gotten together a good mix of toners—he does some isometrics, some calisthenics, and some running classes of exercises in each of his different daily routines. In fact, even though he has a different set of routines for ten sessions during the week, there is always a good combination of three basic exercises for every session. Doctor Franklin even adds a fourth category of exercise for further variation by doing some work with weights as a substitute for some of his morning calisthenics.

Notice also how the Doctor has arranged his routine so that the toners he uses in the morning are done primarily *in an upright position* while in the evening they are done primarily *lying down*. He feels, and I agree, that after sleeping for six or eight hours, *you need to get in an upright position* to exercise. By the same token, after spending a day at whatever job you may do on your feet or sitting, *you need to get flat* to exercise.

Doctor Franklin tells me he's been doing routines similar to the ones I've described with many additional variations for the past 12 years. He says it took him about a year to reach what he considers reasonable tone; and about two years to build up to the numbers of each of the toners he does today. He could, of course, do many more of them—I think he could do sit-ups all day long if he had to, but, as he says, it isn't at all necessary. Why? Simply because what he's accomplishing here is keeping reasonably good tone in his muscles. He's not trying to make himself into a Superman or someone from California's Muscle Beach.

When he first started, Doctor Franklin weighed a flabby 180 pounds, on a rather light five foot, ten inch frame (small boned). Today, he weighs a trim 154 pounds; does not have a loose muscle in his body; looks ten years younger than he did when he started his routines *and he reports he hasn't missed a day's work because of illness in eleven years!*

I'll be talking more about some of Doctor Franklin's toners as we go along in the book, and I've listed many more sets of exercises for physical fitness routines in Chapter 16—all designed to help *you* start on the road to health with physical toning. Don't delay this first step toward dynamic health—the body you save may be your own!

HOW PHYSICAL TONING INCREASES RESISTANCE TO DISEASE

How many athletes have you ever heard of who came down with serious infection? That is, while they were in shape and in good physical condition? The answer is that it is extremely rare.

Why is this? Do you have to be an athlete to achieve this enviable position of impenetrable resistance to disease?

No! You don't have to be an athlete at all. All *you* have to be is in reasonably good physical tone, and that's why delaying *your* toning routines is simply delaying your start to health. That's why you'll want to start in on your routines *now*. Today. Don't be put off—determine just this once that here is one thing you're not going to postpone until next week or next month. There are a few good reasons for getting on the ball with fitness.

START YOUR PROGRAM TODAY FOR EXTRA BENEFITS

Hormones Beefed Up

Hormones are the vital juices produced by the six major sets of glands in your body that regulate virtually every vital process of your body chemistry—and that's a lot of regulating! These invigorating juices bathe every cell in your body at all times. Their concentration depends on what you're doing at any given moment, and on what messages your brain receives from your body's trillions of special cells. Science has found in recent years that the concentration and interdependence of these hormones is more delicate and more subtle than previously imagined—more vital to your general health than ever thought possible.

Physical tone *increases* total hormone production and causes these potent messengers to *stabilize* your body's defenses against infectious disease, stress, wear and tear on joints and muscles, breakdown of cells, aging, and ill health.

It would be simple, you might say, if you could just take the necessary extra hormones. Then you wouldn't have to worry about ill health. Alas! The construction of our bodies isn't so simple, for every time one hormone is increased, one or more other hormones have to be reduced. And maintaining this ever changing balance of hormones can only come as a result of their *natural* production right in your own body. It fact, if hormones are given from outside the body they usually end up causing more damage than good! This is why it is so important to increase their production through natural mechanisms—like physical toning.

I'll be talking more about hormones later in the book. Meanwhile, you can start your own hormone production by doing physical fitness routines twice a day, at least.

New Blood Manufactured

Like anything else that's used up in your body, your blood needs replacing. You might think of it somewhat like the oil in your car that must be drained occasionally and replaced with new oil. Fortunately, your body manufactures its own blood and replaces it automatically.

When you start physical toning, your bone marrow and liver are going to be stimulated to manufacture new blood at a stepped up rate merely because you're now using your blood at a faster rate—you're demanding more of it. New blood brings with it refreshed ability to carry oxygen to, and remove waste products from the body's trillions of cells. With each of your body's cells now able to function more efficiently because oxygen supplies are better and waste doesn't pile up so much, your health automatically gets a tremendous lift through better hormone production (the cells that make hormones need oxygen and waste removing just as any other cells do), better resistance, and better mind function (the cells that make up your mind use more oxygen and need faster elimination of waste than any other cell in your body!).

Better Antibodies Produced

Antibodies are the special chemicals made in your body to neutralize germs and viruses when they invade your body. Antibodies spell the difference between having a strep throat or not having it; between getting pneumonia or not getting it; and between having typhoid fever or tuberculosis or not having it.

I want you to remember this business about antibodies because later I'm going to show you how your mind actually influences the way that your antibodies work. How emotions *do* play a role in your resistance!

Physical fitness does many things for your antibodies. For example, it stimulates new and greater numbers of them to fight disease. Just doing sit-ups, for instance, stimulates your liver every time you make your abdominal muscles pull you up from the floor to the sitting position. Your liver gets "squeezed" each time. This squeezing ejects antibodies into your bloodstream from their storage spots in the liver, and they circulate in your blood seeking out germs and destroying them.

Jogging, as another example, causes your bloodstream to circulate many times faster than usual. This rapidly moving blood courses through your body and increases activity in your lymph glands—the other areas in your body that manufacture antibodies. Just increasing blood circulation surges extra antibodies into your system. Your resistance to disease soars!

LOOKING, FEELING AND ACTING YOUNGER THROUGH PHYSICAL TONING

Even aging is reversed with physical toning! Toning helps eliminate the *clinkers* that pile up in stagnating (unconditioned) cells in your body. When these clinkers are eliminated more efficiently, the cells in your body can function like new again. And when continued physical conditioning prevents the clinkers' formation, your cells retain their youthfulness.

How Julia Got Big Dividends of Youthful Beauty

When I first met Julia D. the uppermost thing on her mind was to have two operations—a face lifting, and an operation to pull up her sagging breasts. She asked me if I could refer her to someone who could do them for her. I said I could but that I thought she could avoid surgery altogether if she were willing to try. Julia laughed and said she'd rather do most anything than undergo surgery, but she thought it was the only way out for her. Sure, she was willing to try. So we started in.

The first thing Julia did was to learn facial isometrics. Twice a day, Julia performed the *clown* routine mentioned earlier. Within only two months, Julia's face began to look more like a 30 year old's than a 55 year old's. The bags disappeared, and the skin beneath her eyes took on a healthy pink luster to replace the dark rings accompanying the bags.

For the sagging breast problem, Julia started a routine of chest and arm isometrics, push-ups and swimming in addition to a weight reduction routine. Within four months, her breasts lost their droopy flab, and became firmly uplifted from their previous droop almost down to her navel. People who knew Julia, including her husband, could hardly believe the changes that followed. All agreed she looked at least ten years younger than before.

Here again, we see in Julia the operation of the body's potential to heal itself—to actually take on the appearance of someone much younger than the chronological age would dictate.

We see the good that can happen to nerves (facial nerves), muscles (the round muscles that surround the eyes), blood vessels (the dark circles beneath the eyes) and skin cells when the clinkers are removed by physical tone.

PHYSICAL TONING AND NUTRITION INSEPARABLE PARTNERS IN TOTAL HEALTH

At this point, I'd like you to refer again to the height-frame-weight tables in Chapter 16. Your aim is to reach ideal weight for your frame and height. *There is nothing that I can think of that will hold you back from health like being overweight!*

Fat creates the following road blocks to dynamic health

1. Sludges blood—retards cell oxygenation and waste elimination.
2. Coats the inside lining of blood vessels—causes blood clots, hardening of arteries, and raises blood pressure that can cause stroke and cornary artery disease.
3. Deposits itself on and around abdominal organs rendering them sluggish and inefficient.
4. Predisposes one to arthritis, lung disease, impotence and cancer.
5. Renders control of health impossible.

These are five excellent reasons to bring your weight under control with physical toning and proper diet *beginning today*.

There are as many diets and nutrition fads that come and go through the years as there are people who like to dream them up. I've found a method so utterly simple and so easy to follow that losing weight properly should be no problem to you whatsoever. A patient I know named Mike V. is so representative of how this can be done that I want to relate his case to you now.

How Fifty-five Year Old Mike Helped Himself to a Great New Life

Mike V. is a fifty-five year old married man who came to me with the following complaints: debilitating arthritis of both hips, knees and ankles; swollen ankles from heart disease; severe shortness of breath; recurrent bouts of bronchitis and pneumonia; and hemorrhoids (piles). Mike was so miserable and so incapacitated from these health problems that he had to quit his job at a local aircraft factory and take a leave of absence. On examining Mike, I also found early diabetes and evidence of artery hardening in addition to high blood pressure.

The one thing you couldn't miss about Mike was that he looked like a walking haystack. He was five foot eight with a medium frame and weighed a whopping 242 pounds! At least 90 pounds over maximum weight for his height and frame!

Poor Mike. In addition to his health woes, he had begun to have side effects from five medicines he'd been taking for some time. He was getting nowhere fast!

Mike was, by this time, a bit mad at the world. He was tired, for instance, of being told he had to do something with his weight. After all, hadn't he tried all the diets? All the fads? Taken all the weight reduction pills without result? I had a long chat with Mike when we first met. I told him I'd accept his case only on the condition that he'd follow my directions to the line. Any deviation and we'd both part company—friends—but we'd part. Finally, he agreed. I think he was so sick and miserable, he'd do almost anything to get better.

First thing I did was to hospitalize him. I probably could have gotten by without doing this, but there was a point I had to drive home to Mike—he had to be convinced that *weight reduction was possible regardless of what his experience had been in the past*. I placed him on a restricted fat and carbohydrate diet *high in protein*. I absolutely forbade visitors until they had been inspected by the floor nurse to make sure no one was bringing poor Mike a fruit basket or other goodies—well meaning, of course, but not conducive to helping Mike's health.

Mike lost 12 pounds in seven days on no medicines—just the diet! And he didn't complain of hunger. When he actually saw that it could be done, he brightened considerably and offered to stick with the diet at home. While in the hospital, Mike was actually able to start physical toning, in spite of his illnesses and disease, mostly through the good graces of the hospital physiotherapist whom I knew to be as great a believer in physical toning as I am.

Of course, Mike wasn't able to do hard calisthenics yet. But he could do most isometrics and could walk and ride a bike short distances. In a two month period, Mike dropped another 30 pounds. His ankle swelling (dropsy) cleared up entirely. Another month saw a 15 pound drop and the complete clearing of signs of heart failure. In two more months, Mike dropped another 20 pounds and at this time his early diabetic state was completely reversed and controlled!

At this time also, Mike was ready and eager to start more difficult toning exercises. He began to do a few push ups and sit-ups every day in addition to isometrics. He began to work with a 30 pound weight, and slowly progressed to a 50 pound bar bell to work out with.

Mike's Health Score with Physical Toning

At the end of seven months Mike had lost a total of 97 pounds! This is faster than I like to see weight lost, but in Mike's case, it was necessary for his health for him to do so.

After a year, lung problems like shortness of breath were complete strangers to Mike. Even his hemorrhoids had resolved themselves with the help of some tips on their care (I'll go into this in a later chapter).

In short, Mike was able to rid himself completely of at least five serious health problems and the only things he used to accomplish this were physical toning and diet!

Today, Mike is a trim 145 pounds. There has been absolutely no recurrence of any of his former states of ill health and he says that he doesn't recall ever having felt so well!

Here is a list of what Mike did for his diet program that will help you get started on your diet program.

1. No calorie counting or weighing of food—he just loaded his plate at meal time with the usual helpings of a balanced diet. Then he removed and replaced *to the serving dish 75 percent of the carbohydrate foods*—potatoes, breads, spaghetti, butter, whole milk, cream, sugar on cereals and in coffee, gravies, salad oils and desserts. He ate only what remained and if he still felt hungry, made up the difference with strictly *protein foods* like meats, fish, poultry, cheeses, vegetables that come in pods (beans, peas, etc.) skim milk, peanut butter. He also utilized the simple reducing diet found in Chapter 16.

2. I made Mike cut his alcohol intake 75 percent—he switched from bourbon and scotch to sherry wine only.

3. He could have all the snacks between meals he wanted as long as they were limited to fruits, carrots, lettuce, salads, crackers, jello, and a special protein recipe snack food designed to alleviate hunger and furnish proper protein nutrition as well. This recipe is found in Chapter 16 for your use.

4. I made Mike reduce the size of his main meals, and get into the habit of eating six smaller meals a day including a bedtime snack. That's all there was to it! Certainly, if Mike can do what he did, so can you and without going in for any fancy fads or super-duper diets. You can do it, that is, *if you remember one important point:* While dieting, always do toning exercises, and always watch your nutrition when toning so that you'll have the best results possible.

SUMMARY

1. If you want to prevent about 75 percent of all the afflictions and diseases that today cripple and debilitate more people than you can imagine, start today with your physical toning and diet routines.
2. The bonuses of physical toning include more and better hormones; more and better antibodies to resist infectious diseases; the reduction of senseless wear and tear on your body; and the toughening and strengthening of your mind!
3. You can do all of these things plus retard the aging process by developing your toning routines at least twice a day: once immediately after arising in the morning and once immediately before going to bed at night.
4. The key point to remember is not to be discouraged by how little you're able to do at first, but to *slowly* and *steadily* increase what you do in the way of exertion over weeks or even months if necessary. Existing disease is no reason to put off developing your routines. How to do this in the face of specific diseases is taken up in sections to follow.
5. The best bet to lose weight is diet plus toning. If you're underweight, toning will automatically bring your weight up through increased nutrition.

3

How to Build New Strength
into Your Heart and Blood Vessels

This chapter concerns heart disease, its prevention and treatment. There is much confusion and myth regarding heart attacks.

I'd like to clear the air on this subject, and show you how to tell if you have heart disease and how it's dealt with once it occurs. Nature has a built-in warning device for protecting the heart. You'll see how this early warning system works and learn how to use it.

Your blood vessels are a prime target for disease of the "wearing down" type. You'll discover how to prevent this from happening to your vessels. Some of you will have already had such trouble. You will be shown how to reestablish dynamic health after such trouble starts. Blood clots and strokes can strike unreasonable fear into the hearts of most people. Both can be prevented and both can be treated satisfactorily in most cases at home as set out in this chapter.

HEADING OFF HEART DISEASE

You're fortunate if you've already begun the basic process of preventing heart and blood vessel disease by doing physical toning routines at least twice every day. This practice increases the tone of your heart muscles as well as stimulating your body to *grow new blood vessels* to carry vital oxygen and energy to your heart muscle which beats 70-80 times every minute, 24 hours a day! *It is these new blood vessels that form as a direct result of your exercising that will spell the difference between having or not having a coronary heart attack and recovering or not recovering if you should have one!*

HOW TO GET OFF THE RISK LIST

The following conditions are known to increase your chances for heart and blood vessel disease:

1. Overweight.
2. Smoking.
3. High blood pressure.
4. Short stocky build.
5. "Pressure job."
6. High blood fats (including cholesterol).

You can rate yourself as follows: Give yourself one point for *each* of the above items if you know that it doesn't apply to you. Give two points if it applies a little and three if any of the items applies a lot. If your total score is above nine, you're a definite cardiac and blood vessel disease risk. Be honest with your scoring—it may save your life or perhaps a lifetime of invalidism, and will spur you on to better health starting today!

Overweight

You're now beginning to see why I devoted an entire chapter to physical toning and ideal weight control (Chapter 2). If there has been any doubt in your mind in understanding the essence of Chapter 2, I suggest you read it again—*40 percent of all heart and blood vessel disease would disappear in the United States if the single factor of being overweight were eliminated!*

Consult again the height-weight-frame tables in Chapter 16. Consult the reducing diets listed there as well. *Get with* weight control and physical toning today if you value your healthful life.

Smoking

If you smoke more than two packs of cigarettes a day, you're a heavy smoker; if between one and two packs, a moderate smoker; and if less than a pack daily, a light smoker. Much has been said about smoking and disease and much more has been written. The truth is, with smoking, *it's the amount you smoke,* not the fact that you smoke. Strive to become a light smoker—a half pack or less a day. You don't have to give up; *just cut down.* Cigars and pipes appear to be harmless insofar as heart and blood vessel disease is concerned, but I'll have more to say about them later.

Blood Pressure Problems

Blood pressure can be tricky. Although it's not impossible to record your own blood pressure, it's best to let someone else do it who has had experience using the blood pressure cuff. There are two readings with blood pressure—one written above the line and one written below the line. For instance, 130/80 is referred to as 130 over 80. In this example, the 130 is the systolic reading—the pressure inside your arteries when your heart contracts. The 80 is the diastolic reading—the pressure inside your arteries when your heart relaxes.

The diastolic reading is the more important since it shows the pressure in your artery during its relaxed phase. The more rigid an artery when relaxed the tighter its muscle coating, and the tighter the muscle coating, the greater the chance of its causing trouble—coronaries, strokes and clots.

The first line of attack on blood pressure is *weight control!* Yet another of many reasons for getting your weight close to ideal for very few cases of high blood pressure among people of ideal weight need to be treated with medicine to bring it down.

One blood pressure reading does not mean much. Four or five readings taken at weekly intervals over four to six weeks are much more accurate for a blood pressure estimate. It's normal, for example, for your blood pressure to rise during any exertion. But it drops right back down again when you stop exerting. There is nothing harmful in this rise. Being tense and upset makes blood pressure go up. When calm again, it should come right back down.

Body-build

People who are fairly short, stockily built (heavily muscled plus overweight) and who tend to get little exercise are peculiarly prone to heart and blood vessel disease. I realize you can't pick your inheritance, but you *can* lose weight and start toning routines. You can't change your basic build, but you *can be tougher in getting the other five high risk factors under control.*

Pressure on the Job

Not enough attention in my opinion, has been paid to this fact of being under constant and continual high stress on the job. I mean by this people who worry constantly about getting a job done, or about what someone else is going to think about the way they do their work, coupled with having to constantly be concerned about deadlines in their job. It's been shown that such people are in jeopardy from heart and blood vessel disease. The only way I know to avoid this factor is to be transferred to another job where you don't feel the edge of pressure so much or where deadlines day in and day out are not the business of the day.

Blood Fats

If you're overweight, you can be sure that your blood fats—cholesterol and others—are too high. You don't need to be tested to know this. Your weight must be brought under control.

Even after weight control, there are some people who are still high in cholesterol and other fats. If this is the case, a low cholesterol diet is in order plus perhaps one of the newer medicines that lowers the levels of blood fats.

It doesn't take much time or trouble to drop into a laboratory or to a hospital outpatient department on the way to work some morning to have this testing done. Short of this, consult Chapter 16 and follow the low cholesterol diet you'll find there. You can combine this diet quite easily with any reducing diet for double safety.

DOES ALCOHOL HURT?

In the case of heart and blood vessel disease, either extreme with alcohol can be harmful. This is best illustrated by the cases of two people, Jenny and Bill.

Jenny Throws the Habit

Jenny was an alcoholic, and had been one for ten years. She was reluctant to admit it, but I finally pulled it out of her one day in the office. The clue came from recurrent ulcer symptoms even though she was on a strict diet and medicine control for them. This is always a suspicious element with someone who drinks too much.

Jenny had enough liver damage from her excess alcohol to have started trouble. Her liver wasn't able to break down waste products that normally accumulate in the body. When these built up enough, they started kidney trouble. Jenny had a mild weight problem, but correcting this didn't cure the kidney problem. What did cure it, finally, was the elimination of alcohol from Jenny's life. This was difficult and she did it primarily herself with the aid of *Alcoholics Anonymous.* When her liver healed, it once again began to take care of the waste products and her kidney function returned to normal.

Bill's Problem

Bill was just the opposite. He worked under a head of steam all day long day in and day out for years. He'd never taken a drink of anything in his life on religious grounds. After a difficult struggle with Bill's elevated blood pressure—primarily from being over-weight and under too much constant pressure at work—I finally talked him into making it a habit on arriving home to take from two to four ounces of sherry wine before dinner. It worked like a charm. Bill was able to discontinue all medicines and hasn't had a tranquilizer since, though he lived on them before health control was reached.

As a result, Bill hasn't had blood pressure difficulties for more than eight years, and has interrupted his nervous state with the proper use of one of the best tranquilizers I know of—a glass of wine!

HEART ATTACK—IS IT THE END?

The human body's ability to heal itself is nothing short of fantastic. True, the results aren't always perfect, but when you stop to consider all the things the body can do for itself, you can't help but marvel.

Let's say you're like a man I know named John R., age 54, married, and who has had his first coronary attack. I'd like to tell you what happened to John and how I'd have done it differently had I been John's physician from the start. It wasn't until some time after his heart attack that John came to me, so what followed was already history when I met him.

You Can Recover Just Like John

John, it seems, was stricken with his coronary at work, taken to a hospital and immediately plunked into an intensive care unit—a relatively new part of a hospital concerned with the care of the seriously and critically ill. Yes, the doctor told John, he'd had a heart attack alright. Not a big one, but nevertheless a coronary occlusion that started as most do—a sudden, severe, crushing sensation under the breastbone; difficulty getting in a breath of air; profuse sweating; and spreading of the chest pain up to the left shoulder and down the inside of the left upper arm.

Now the current scientific rules and regulations say that such an individual must remain almost motionless, and flat in bed for three weeks. This is where I'd first disagree with the popular notion. John was forced to remain immobilized in bed for three weeks after he got out of the intensive care section even though on the fifth day, most of his pain and discomfort was gone and he was becoming very fidgety, confined as he was to bed.

Instead of sizing up what seemed to be a different situation in John's case, he was given strong sedatives to insure he stayed immobilized and in bed. In short, John was forced to remain in his mummified condition with the threat that if he didn't, he might kill himself with the slightest exertion.

It was at this point that John became so scared of his heart and what *might* happen that he became a prisoner of his own fears—a psychological cripple, paralyzed by what might happen if he didn't toe the line.

Your Post Heart Attack Schedule

My own view is that *most* heart attacks such as this need not be treated with such strict immobility, but that, barring complications, certain activities can be started on the third or fourth day. Naturally, no one thinks the patient ought to be doing calisthenics, but changing position and going to the bathroom on other than a bed pan (the most devilish invention of the twentieth century) seems to be in order.

The point is, that when John arrived home during the fourth week after his attack, he was so worried about a catastrophe that he sat frozen in a chair, though perfectly able to move about and do essential things for himself. And he sat, and sat, and sat. John's wife waited on him hand and foot, even more concerned than John that the slightest exertion might bring on another, and perhaps fatal calamity. In my view, John should have been moving freely about the house, going to the bathroom by himself and doing a few extra things to help his wife at this time.

As it was, after six weeks had passed and John's heart healing process had long since completed itself, he was still an armchair invalid. And nothing anyone could say would get it out of his head that it was perfectly safe to start getting back into the swing of things again. He put on more weight. His muscles became soft and flabby from disuse. His mental attitude deteriorated with each passing day. He aged about ten years in six weeks!

How John Responded to Common Sense Health Control

There are far too many problems like John's. Maybe not as pronounced, but problems even so. In going over the risk table I listed earlier in this chapter, I estimated John to score 13—a moderately severe risk for cardiac or blood vessel disease. With a little doing, John could easily have forced this count below 9, taking him out of the high risk category. But all that was past. Here he was—well on his way to becoming a permanent invalid. Sound like health under good control? Definitely not!

My first contact with John came with a visit to his house because his physician had become ill himself and asked me to look in on him. I couldn't believe what I found. And to make matters worse, John was beginning to have signs of phlebitis in the veins of one leg as a result of his sitting in a chair so long all day! And that's all John needed—something else to complicate the picture!

I began to explore the elements of health control with John. He was horrified at the idea of getting up, walking around the block, or starting physical toning routines. He'd never bothered with them before his heart attack and the idea of doing anything so drastic at this time was simply out of the question as far as John was concerned.

I finally told him that if he didn't start it and start it soon, he'd never get out of his chair again. He said he'd wait to hear from his own doctor. And he did. Trouble is he waited too long—he developed acute thrombosis in one leg, a clot broke off and traveled to his lungs where trouble started that proved much worse than his original heart attack.

A Schedule for Heart Attack Patients

Here is a schedule that most heart attack patients can tolerate. John should have been on it.

1. *First week:* Sit in chair in hospital room, go to bathroom, (no straining from constipation and plenty of fluids—laxatives beforehand will prevent this

from being a problem). Deep breathing and leg exercises (discussed later in this chapter).

2. *Second week:* Out of bed for stroll; visit friends in lobby; leg exercises; weight reduction if necessary.

3. *Third week:* Fully ambulatory; to physiotherapy department of hospital for carefully supervised leg, abdominal, and arm exercises.

4. *At home:* Graduated and *careful* toning routine started, weight control started, mental conditioning started. Appropriate diet continued and enforced.

If You've Had Heart Difficulties, Remember These Points

1. In any coronary attack, the die is cast in the first 24 hours—either your heart has the capacity to recover or it doesn't. If the latter, nothing will prevent the inevitable. If the former (usual case), then you've every reason to begin to think about and do those things that experience proves will *reduce the risk of another attack* and that will return you to a perfectly normal life again. Perhaps a much better life than you've had at any time in the past!

2. Nature has provided your heart with an early warning device I'll discuss a little later. Rely on it. Depend on it. Don't let yourself be done out of an active, useful and healthy life.

3. When you arrive home, start things off *slowly* at first. Don't leap back into your previous habits. Think about Chapter 2 first. Find out what must be done to reduce your risks and aim to accomplish these things first. Ask questions of your doctor. If you don't understand the answer, ask again until you do.

ANGINA PECTORIS

Angina means heart pain. It usually occurs beneath your breastbone, as in the case of a coronary attack, but it isn't nearly so overwhelming or uncomfortable. The pain may be to the left of your breastbone and may spread to your shoulder, neck, jaw or arm on the left side. *It occurs when you've overdone yourself, physically.* It is the built-in early warning device I mentioned a bit ago. Pay attention to it. It signals you've reached your physical limit! It lets up when you rest.

June Thought She Was "Done For"

June W. thought she was having a heart attack when, during the course of her physical toning routine and before she'd lost much weight, she noticed deep, knife-like pain beneath her left breast. It seemed to travel to her shoulder as well. She was surprised nine months later when she could do three times the physical exertion *after reducing her weight to ideal level* without any discomfort or chest distress whatsoever. June was experiencing angina of effort— her heart was telling her it wasn't time to do that much exertion with that much weight yet to be lost.

How Ralph Dealt with Chest Pains

Ralph K. called me one day to report he was sitting in a lounge chair in his backyard when he felt pain in the left side of his chest—the side of his chest covered by his arm as it hung by his side. When he moved or breathed in deeply, it hurt worse; when he remained still, it was quite mild.

Ralph didn't have angina. Why? In the first place, the distress came on while Ralph was resting—angina usually comes on during exertion or strain. Angina hurts just as much if you're not moving after it starts and breathing doesn't affect its intensity. Ralph was having pain from a nerve running along the underside of one of his ribs—probably brought on by lack of physical tone and the stretched out position he was in at the time.

Angina as a Warning Bell

Whether you've never had heart trouble before or after you've had a coronary like John's, angina can be relied upon to tell you when to *stop whatever it is you're doing and rest*. And it can warn you to stop your physical activity short of the beginning of chest pain next time you do physical activity, whether it's walking or doing toning routines.

HEART ROUTINES

The most common heart medicines are of the digitalis group and of the nitroglycerin type. Digitalis is used when the heart muscle fibers need help with their contraction and with certain irregularities of heart rhythm. Nitroglycerin or a derivative is taken to prevent or stop angina—heart pain.

The fact that you take either of these groups of drugs should not deter you from practicing those teachings that remove you from the high risk of heart and blood vessel diseases. In fact, physical toning as set out in this book, done properly, and coupled with weight control, may well enable your heart to do with less of these medicines or may even allow you to be perfectly comfortable and healthy without them. You need to keep in close touch with the practitioner who prescribed these drugs—he is best qualified to guide you on proper dose and frequency.

These Rules of Thumb Will Guide You if You're on Heart Medicines

1. Don't take any other medicine of any kind until you've checked it out with your doctor who prescribed the heart medicine.
2. Take heart medicine *exactly as prescribed*—don't lower or raise the dose without advice.
3. If you feel the medicine makes you sick, check with whomever prescribed it for advice.
4. Most medicines like nitroglycerin taken for angina cause giddiness or dizzyness as a side reaction. This isn't harmful unless it persists for a long time.
5. Remember that getting control of your health may change the need for heart medicine—check with your medical consultant at regular intervals if you feel you need less medicine.

FLUTTERS AND PALPITATIONS

There is no end to the way your nerves can play tricks on you—make you think things are going on in your body when nothing really major is going on. Your heart is a favorite site for such *tricks.*

How Betty Overcame Palpitations

When Betty I. called me, she thought she was having a heart attack because her heart was turning *flip-flops.* When I examined her during a flip-flop attack, I found her heart rate and rhythm quite regular and normal. Betty was tense, nervous and an extreme worrier. Her nerves were making her think that her heart action was irregular. Betty learned to concentrate while resting during such attacks. She simply concentrated on relaxing completely and feeling no more flip-flops. She eventually learned to stop the flip flops in about five minutes and remains in good health today.

How Harold Beat Flutters and Fainting

Harold E., on the other hand, complained he was beginning to have fainting spells for the first time in his 58 years. He said they occurred two or three times a week and were always preceded by a feeling of dizzyness and sweating. Then he'd simply slump over on a chair or lounge when he felt a spell coming on. Harold did indeed have an irregular heart rhythm—a special kind that threw his heart off timing. Harold's irregularities were cured with a single medicine designed to counteract the irregular beats. His fainting spells stopped permanently and have not returned.

How to Test and Control Palpitations

Most palpitations are like Betty's. They're harmless pranks being played by your nerves. To really tell if your heartbeat rhythm is off, sit down, place the tip of one of your fingers on the artery you see pulsating at your wrist or at your temple. Normal rhythm is an equally spaced succession of pulses. If the rhythm isn't normal, you'll notice a series of beats followed by pauses that you can easily feel, or you'll feel extra beats between the usual ones. It's always wise to get a professional opinion if you feel irregularities in your pulse.

In Betty's case, she learned to relax and to channel emotion to control her palpitations. She learned that physical exercise during an emotional upheaval—such as when she felt herself getting angry or depressed—was an excellent way to blow off steam as well as prevent palpitations. This, together with working on other parts of health control finally stopped the palpitations altogether.

HARD ARTERIES AND VARICOSE VEINS

It's not too late to start enjoying life even though you may have hardening of the arteries. The first thing on your schedule to start up the road to health is to begin physical and mental control. As you begin your toning routines, you may notice, as a patient of mine, Mac N. did, that trouble is starting in one of your legs. Mac was walking, cycling and playing golf and enjoying it until he noticed that with progressively less and less exertion, he had severe, deep pains develop in the calf muscle of his right leg. The pain would disappear after rest, but came back again and again. Mac suspected something very wrong and he was correct. Examination showed the major artery to his right leg was so narrowed down that the demand for oxygen and energy brought on by his exercising was too much for the hardened artery to supply. His calf muscle pained from this lack of essential energy and oxygen.

There was a time, and not too long ago, that such a case would dictate a reduction of physical activitiy or invite disaster. Mac was fortunate because our colleagues, the surgeons, have developed ways and means of correcting such an unfortunate situation. The surgeons in Mac's case removed the hardened portion of the leg artery and substituted a special plastic tube in its place.

Today, Mac can do any and all physical exercise he wishes without pain or discomfort in his leg. And the technique of the surgeon isn't limited to leg arteries. Surgeons today can, if necessary, replace even a large portion of the aorta, the largest artery in your body—the one that leads out of your heart and supplies virtually all the blood to the rest of the body's major artery trunks!

If the hardening process happens to cause an arterial weak spot with the production of a *balloon* (like a weak spot in an inflated car inner tube—a bulging out of the artery) surgeons can usually remove this balloon and restore the artery to normal again.

Varicose Veins: What to Do About Them

Varicose veins are the most common affliction of blood vessels—and the easiest to control! They can occur almost anywhere, but seem to prefer the legs. Varicose veins are simply veins that have lost their elastic connective tissue coating surrounding the thin muscle wall of the vein. This loss allows the veins to pop up and protrude through the skin as twisting bluish knots of veins. When varicose veins develop, they're usually unsightly, cause legs to ache, and the skin to feel burny and itchy. Sometimes ulcers on the skin develop around varicose veins.

Varicose veins can start at any age—they're common in young people after childbirth, but generally come on after middle age.

A Program to Deal with Varicose Veins of Your Legs

1. When you're not sitting down, *keep moving.* Standing around without moving your legs is the single *worst* thing for varicose veins in your legs!

2. When you're sitting down, *elevate both legs onto another chair, stool, or whatever,* so that your legs are at least even or slightly elevated above waist level.

3. If varicose veins are fairly large or widespread on your legs, both legs should be kept wrapped with elastic supports or bandages during the day. These are the rolled cloth and rubber dressings with two or three metal fasteners attached to them that you wrap snugly around your foot, ankle,

lower and even upper leg, if necessary, and which stretch to fit snugly when pulled as they are applied.

It's important to start your wrap at that section of your foot where your toes join your foot and work upward toward your knee. Aim for snugness—not too tight or too loose. Then use the fasteners to hold the upper end of the wrap in place. If these get lost or fall off, a safety pin or two will do just as well.

4. Keep the skin around varicose veins well-moistened and lubricated with any good emolient like hand lotion or face cream. Rub in thoroughly three times a day.

5. If you're going out and don't want the elastic bandages to show, purchase a good set of elastic hose—don't use cheap ones, they're no good. Be certain they fit well and use them!

6. If the pain and discomfort progress or ulcers form on your skin from varicose veins, surgery for their removal may be indicated. This is not major surgery, and done properly, cures them once and for all.

Varicose veins can occur in areas other than your legs. If they appear in your rectum, for example, they're called piles or hemorrhoids (discussed in a later chapter), if in your nose, they cause nose bleeds; and if on the male testicle, they're called varicoceles. But they all mean the same, namely, that the veins have lost their normal support and protrude through to the surface.

Veins that are simply visible through the skin—do not actually protrude, in other words—are not varicose veins, cause no trouble, and should not be cause for any alarm or treatment.

BLOOD CLOTS AND PHLEBITIS

When there develops tenderness, swelling and redness around the vicinity and along the course of a leg or arm vein, it's called thrombo-phlebitis—shortened to just phlebitis. This is not the dangerous complication that you might think but is simply an inflamnation of the lining of the vein. It can be cured by hot moist packs in the form of hand towels soaked in very warm water and wrapped around the extremity and well above and below the areas of redness and tenderness. This can be done for 30-40 minutes four times a day until the signs have gone. The towels should be replaced as they are felt to cool and be replaced by hot ones.

Blood Clots Do Not Result from Phlebitis

A patient named Mavis W. was recuperating from minor surgery in the hospital and suddenly developed chest pain, fever, difficulty in breathing and spitting up of blood. She had developed a blood clot in the deep veins of her leg, it had broken off in the circulation, and traveled to her lungs. Mavis allowed herself to become lazy during her surgical recovery: *She had neglected her health control—had failed to start exercising the day after surgery.* The blood in her legs had pooled there and become stagnant from inactivity and a clot had formed.

Preventing Deep Vein Phlebitis

Fortunately for Mavis, she recovered with proper treatment but the sad part is, the trouble might have been prevented if Mavis had been doing what she should have. The following two simple devices will usually prevent blood clots from forming during any period when you may be inactive (such as following surgery; illness at home; long auto trips) for longer than usual.

1. Every hour all the leg and foot muscles should be stretched as far as they can be. The toes forcibly curled up then straightened out; the entire foot turned inwardly, then outwardly as far as possible several times; then flexed upwardly and downwardly as far as possible several times (this flexes the lower leg muscles); the knees flexed, then extended as far as possible several times; the thighs flexed at the hip, rotated in a circle at the hip and forced outwardly to the side, then inwardly toward the middle several times. All muscles firmly contracted during each period.
2. Every hour, you should take in ten breaths of air as deeply as you can force your lungs to suck in; then force out every wisp of air inside your lungs. At the end of ten breaths, you should forcibly cough several times.

The clots that form in the deep veins of the foot and leg cannot be felt (until it's too late) and can't be seen like surface phlebitis can. It is important for you to forestall any such trouble by using the above maneuvers whenever you find yourself inactive, for whatever reasons. Even standing around on a job all day long should be interrupted at hourly intervals for these toning procedures. Blood clots can be prevented. Don't neglect your foot and leg toning to prevent them!

PREVENTING STROKES

Strokes are caused by blood vessel leaks or clots inside the head. All the things I've talked about regarding blood vessel disease thus far apply as well for blood vessels inside your head. When a clot forms inside a brain blood vessel or when a weak spot in a brain vessel gives way, a *stroke* is said to have occurred.

Little Strokes

This name is applied to disease of the very small blood vessels in your brain. A little stroke may also involve a larger vessel—such as with a short episode of reduced blood flow to a part of the brain. In any event, small strokes may go almost unnoticed and may happen frequently without detection. Usually, something happens—a feeling of strangeness, a little dizziness, some trouble with your balance, a short period where spoken words don't come as easy as usual—any number of short-lived signs that usually clear up entirely. Such signs usually mean something is going on that shouldn't be, but they rarely cause permanent or serious damage. The same rules apply to the "big" strokes as far as activity goes.

Big Strokes

This means trouble in one of the large major arteries inside your head—one that supplies vital blood and oxygen to a large area of the brain. There may be unconsciousness following a severe headache; all kinds of eye symptoms such as partial loss of vision; loss of ability to speak; and the like. The side of the body opposite the side of the brain involved may become weak or even paralyzed.

But it should be remembered that virtually all these signs are reversible in the large percentage of cases. They can and do disappear—sometimes not completely, but enough so that perfectly normal function may be regained in most instances.

The key to prevention of strokes is to keep your blood pressure as close to normal as possible, to keep weight down as near to the ideal as possible, and to reduce fats and cholesterol to low levels. This ring a familiar bell? It should. It is exactly what I've been talking about in the previous two chapters! If you've had a stroke already, *this is all the more reason to master completely the material in the first two chapters.*

How Dan Applied Common Sense Health and Is Now Well

A man I'll call Dan had his first major stroke at age 59. The stroke (sometimes called a CVA—cerebrovascular accident) left him speechless, completely paralyzed on the right side, unable to completely control his bladder and rectum, and without ability to move any of the muscles on the left side of his face.

The following shows what simple rehabilitation and health principles can do if properly applied as they were in Dan's case:

1. Dan lived in the country, so all treatment was done at home, mostly at first by his wife. First a catheter—a rubber or plastic tube—was placed into his bladder so that his bladder wouldn't empty on the bed clothes. A catheter like this one can be controlled by anyone with five minutes of practice.

2. Liquids and very soft feedings were started (he had difficulty swallowing and with half his face and jaw paralyzed, he couldn't chew properly) six times a day utilizing protein powder dissolved in skim milk or juices; egg nogs; jellos; junkets; and custards along with plenty of water so his body could continue properly to eliminate wastes. For a time, Dan's wife had to place a plastic stomach tube down his gullet in order to feed him. In ten days, Dan could swallow well enough on his own without the tube.

3. I taught Dan's wife the technique of asking all of Dan's paralyzed muscles to do some work at least three times a day.

> *For his face:* Simple massage was enough—anything to stimulate the muscles and nerves, stroking and rubbing the muscles using a lotion to moisten the fingers doing the massage for five or six minutes.
>
> *For his neck:* Grasping the back of his head with her hand and flexing it so that his chin was brought down to his chest several times.
>
> *For his shoulder.* Grasping his left arm and simply rotating it around in a wide circle several times and then drawing his arm up at the side so that it was brought up and over his head each time.
>
> *For his arm:* Flexing and extending at the elbow several times: twisting at the elbow, first palm up, then palm down.
>
> *For his hand:* Flexion and extending hand at wrist several times; curling up each finger so as to make a fist several times, then straightening all of them out again.
>
> *For his leg:* Rotating his leg at the hip several times; drawing up his thigh toward his abdomen and back down again several times; bending and straightening the lower leg at the knee joint several times; flexing and straightening the foot at the ankle joint several times; and curling all the toes.

On the third day following his stroke, Dan was sitting up on the side of his bed six times a day with his wife's help. He was doing exercises with small weights using his unaffected right arm and leg as well as doing isometrics. He was doing, in other words, just what you should be doing in your physical toning routines!

Within three weeks, Dan was getting some movement back into his paralyzed arm and leg and could move some of his small face muscles on his own. The toning was beginning to do just what I mentioned it would do in Chapter 2. Energy was traveling up the nerves to damaged brain cells by means of his own and his wife's constant application of the basic rules of toning. It was paying off—he was overcoming the effects of a serious stroke, and was preventing his useless muscles from shrinking through disuse!

Dan was walking with help by five weeks. He was controlling his bladder by eight weeks and was able to manage his life completely on his own.

Today, the only way you can tell Dan had a stroke at all is by the slight droop of the left side of his mouth when he smiles. There is no sign otherwise! And because Dan has removed himself from the high risk heart and blood vessel list, he will probably not have another stroke. The only medicine Dan takes is four tablets a day to control his blood pressure which was high to begin with but now remains normal. Small price to pay for the way back to health!

SUMMARY

1. Heart diseases and blood vessel damage can be prevented. Mastering principles of weight control, high risk factors, and physical fitness are ways you can prevent this trouble.
2. Get yourself off the high risk heart and blood vessel disease list today by following the guide to prevention of coronary and stroke problems.
3. Nerves play a great role in many heart rhythm difficulties. You can overcome most of them by utilizing the principles of health control.
4. Once a coronary or stroke has occurred, rehabilitation back to normal and your continuing health depends absolutely on health control principles.
5. Any and all medicines used for heart or blood vessel disease should be prescribed, followed along, and changed only by your medical advisor.

4

How to Revitalize Your Blood
for Exhilarating Health

Blood is the essence of your life and you should know how to keep it in tone. We've just looked at the heart and blood vessels, the permanent home for blood. You will now see how the two are in constant equilibrium and how they are kept that way for good health.

Besides carrying vital oxygen and energy to the trillions of cells in your body, blood has five other major functions: resistance to disease, body thermostat, master communicator, nutrition carrier and waste disposer. In this section you'll discover how to keep each of these functions in top condition, and how you can improve them if they seem inadequate.

Blood is life. Therefore it pays to know what blood does and how to keep it humming along with fresh vitality and power. This section will cover this vital function.

HOW YOUR BLOOD FUNCTIONS AS AN ORGAN

Blood is another of your body's vital organs. It's composed of several specialized tissues just like any other organ. The only difference between blood and most other organs is that it is constantly in motion—moving vital chemicals and nutrients in and out of every single cell in your body.

What gives blood its motion is your heart. With each contraction, your heart pumps blood through your arteries under pressure, insuring that all your cells are bathed in life-giving substances.

Red Cells Carry Your Vital Oxygen

Red blood cells are what gives blood its unique color. They have

63

a double purpose: To bind oxygen they pick up as they pass through your lungs, and to bind carbon dioxide (the end point of all human metabolism) as they pass near the cells.

The unique chemical, called hemoglobin, makes up the bulk of red blood cells. This remarkable chemical is able to attract the oxygen you breathe into your lungs and then give it back up to the cells of your body. As soon as the oxygen is given up, the waste product of the cells, carbon dioxide, is immediately attracted to red blood cells and it is given up into the lungs and exhaled with each breath.

How You Can Benefit by Increasing Your Red Cells

You can increase your red blood cells by stimulating their turnover—by making your body produce more new red cells. Where do red blood cells come from? From the inside of your bones—from the bone marrow. The average life of a red blood cell is between six and eight days. When they're worn out, they go to the spleen where they are broken down to bile and sent to the liver for storage and use in digestion—a remarkable recycling process, wouldn't you agree?

To produce more red cells, you need to increase the amount of exercise you do. In other words, by starting the routines I talked about in Chapter 2, you've already begun to increase your red cell production. Exercise hastens the recycling of worn-out red cells as well.

The one essential ingredient in making new red cells is iron. You get iron from protein in your diet. You can also take iron directly, a topic I'll discuss further later in this chapter. But if you have plenty of protein in your diet, you usually don't need extra iron.

How Blood Serum Revitalizes Your Body

Blood serum is the liquid part of blood—the carrier of all the cells (including red cells, white cells, blood-clotting cells), all your body's essential nutritional substances (including protein, carbohydrate and fat), hormones, and a list of chemicals that would fill a volume!

How efficient is serum? It's hard to believe, but if someone were to inject a substance into one of the veins in your arm, and this substance happened to have a bitter taste, you would taste the bitterness in about six or seven seconds! In other words, the serum would carry the substance through your arm and into the right side of your heart, then through your lungs, then back to the left side of your heart, then into the main artery of your neck, then into several branching arteries until it reaches the artery to your tongue—all in six or seven seconds!

Stirring up Your Serum

You can make your serum more efficient by keeping your circulation stirred up by taking frequent breaks during the day to exercise, even if it's just a walk out in the fresh air; and by learning to breathe deeply of fresh air—to force out stale air that always resides in your lungs and suck in new vital oxygen to replace it. And you can eat a proper diet with plenty of protein, moderate carbohydrate and small amounts of fat.

HOW MILLIE THREW OFF THE YOKE OF SLUGGISH SERUM

I've known hundreds of patients like Millie E., for example, who seemed to have trouble during the middle of the day, especially in colder weather, with feeling "loggy" and listless. When I talk to people like Millie I find that they are busily at work in an office or in their homes when this extreme fatigue and lethargy hits. Their blood is stagnant and is sludgy—all Millie needed to do was to stop whatever it is that she happened to be doing every couple of hours, go to an open window and take in a dozen forced deep breaths and then blow out as much air from her lungs as possible. When appropriate, I advised Millie to take a walk outside or search out an empty room, open the window and do some jogging in place, push-ups or isometrics in the presence of fresh air.

Millie was amazed at the difference. She found out how to revitalize her blood as a matter of course each and every day. Her lethargy and listless feelings were promptly cured.

I'm certain you've noticed how invigorating it is to go out into a cold wintry blast and shovel the snow or just take a short walk. This is because your blood is supercharged when you do. It's stirred up and replenished with vital oxygen and energy, and it serves you more efficiently.

HOW TO KEEP YOUR BLOOD AND VESSELS
FUNCTIONING SMOOTHLY

Since your blood and the vessels in which it's contained are inseparable partners throughout life, enhancing the function of one will necessarily increase the efficiency of the other. I discussed your heart and blood vessels in the previous chapter. Let's look further at this relationship.

How Vessel Walls Affect Your Health

Outside blood vessel walls are mainly muscle, and are considerably thicker in arteries than in veins. With each contraction of your heart, the arteries expand. When the heart relaxes, so do your arteries.

The inside lining of your blood vessels are very thin membranes. They're quite sensitive to what's going on in the blood as it constantly flows over them. If there should be damage (as from a cut or scratch) a special chain reaction occurs between this membrane and the blood that forms a clot to stop any bleeding or oozing that may occur from the vessel. Nature's way of preventing loss of vital blood!

Blood Fats Are Dangerous to Your Health

The inside lining membrane is particularly susceptible to large fat globs that may float about in your blood. The lining traps such globs from time to time and eventually, if the globs are plentiful as in a fat person, they form a plaque—a collection of globs which eventually grows until the inside of the artery narrows down. *This is what starts the events that lead to coronary heart disease and strokes, and may cut off blood supply to an arm or leg.*

Final Health of Your Cells Is Governed by Capillaries

Blood vessels vary in size from as big as your wrist (the aorta) to microscopic size. The microscopic size blood vessels are the last of the branches of blood vessels. They're so small that only a single file of red cells can travel down them. It's in these capillaries that the nutrients leave your blood and the wastes pass into them. The serum or any part of it may pass entirely outside the capillaries directly to the cells, then return again.

Capillaries are found in profusion everywhere in your body. If you stretched out these tiny tubes, they'd extend for hundreds of miles! They are rich in nerve endings that reduce or increase their openness or closedness in any given area. When your fingers get cold, it's because the capillaries are closed down; a feeling of warmth in your skin means many more capillaries have been opened. It's also possible that the capillaries can be opened so wide as to allow both red cells and white cells (discussed later in the chapter) to escape their confines.

The fact, then that your blood has constant access to literally every cell in your body means that the condition of your blood is crucial to your health.

HOW TO KEEP YOUR BLOOD VESSELS SURGING WITH VIGOROUS HEALTH

This list of points will enable you to help your blood and blood vessels maintain their vital working relationship:

1. Be certain that you take in plenty of iron in your diet. This means plenty of protein. And iron, if for some reason your protein intake falls below par. One iron tablet a day is all your system can absorb—any more than this will be wasted and unnecessary.

2. Practice good daily physical toning, including breathing breaks.

3. If you don't get plenty of fruits and fruit juices, take in extra Vitamin C. This vitamin helps maintain the vitality of the inside lining of blood vessels and promotes the absorption of iron.

4. Reduce fats to a minimum in your diet. Use *unsaturated* (margarine) spreads, vegetable cooking oils and salad dressings. Eliminate butter, cream, and saturated cooking oils (lard and other solid preparations).

5. Although your heart pumps your blood through your arteries, the return of blood through the vein system back to your lungs and heart depends on *physical (muscular) activity entirely. Start physical toning today!*

HOW TO DEVELOP BLOOD'S OTHER FUNCTIONS TO PERFECTION

For Disease Resistance

Your blood is the battleground for germ invasion. Consider the following sequence of events:

1. Your body is invaded by a germ—maybe a virus causing a cold, maybe a bacteria causing a strep throat. What actually happens more often is that the virus or strep is there all the time, your body defenses having kept it under control.

2. Blood carries *invader* to special tissues that *measure it up* for the correct antibody to knock out the germ. The specially made up antibody is carried by the blood to the germ and applied to it, neutralizing it.

3. Special chemicals elaborated by tissues (cells) tell blood to concentrate white cells at certain spots. White cells surround and digest germs.

4. Proteins needed for antibodies are carried in the blood. Antibodies are carried indefinitely in the blood after they're made to take care of future invasions by a similar germ.

HOW BILLY AND MOLLY FARED WITH RESISTANCE PROBLEMS

I've seen literally hundreds of Billy's and Molly's, two youngsters each with a slightly different problem of interference with blood resistance problems.

Billy L.

He is a three year old from whom somebody decided to remove his tonsils on the basis of two or three previous strep throats. Over the next four years, Billy had bronchopneumonia six different times. Why? Because the tonsils are functional against infections that enter the body through the nose and mouth at this early age.

Although the tonsils can become pussy and infected many times at this age, they are also part of the specialized tissue to which blood delivers germs to be "measured" for antibodies. If they're gone, they can't very well do this function. So, when the germs get into the nose and mouth, they progress down the breathing tract and can cause more serious pneumonia.

> *LESSON:* Try *not* to remove tonsils until after seven or eight years of age even though they may be infected a lot and need treatment. After this age, other tissues take over the protective function, and the blood has by this time saved up sufficient antibodies to fight off such infections adequately.

Molly R.

She is a four year old in a Midwestern college town. Her parents ran her to the doctor with each and every sniffle. At these times, she would get penicillin or one of the other antibiotics. As a consequence, Molly grew into her teens going through misery with one infection after another—colds and virus infections all the time and a weak and frail constitution. In addition, she became allergic to penicillin and can no longer have it for any reason under penalty of severe allergic consequences.

LESSON: Antibiotics are *not* needed for virus infections. They do no good (viruses are not the least affected by penicillin); they retard the body's ability to make its own antibodies; and you run the serious risk of developing allergies to antibiotics if they are taken for every sign or symptom. Give your blood a chance. That's what it's for!

Nor do all bacterial infections need the benefit of the *miracle* antibiotics.

HOW YOU CAN BENEFIT FROM JACK'S EXPERIENCE WITH INFECTION

Jack V. developed a large boil on his posterior. When I saw him he asked for "something to kill it off."
Here is what Jack really needed and it cured his trouble completely:

1. Local application of hot moist packs four times a day for 30 minutes. As the washcloth he was using cooled down, he was to replace it with a hot one.
2. This brought the boil to a head in two days time. It began to drain out the pus by itself. He kept a clean loose dressing over it between hot moist pack applications *which were kept up at an increased rate now that the boil was draining.*
3. In a week's time, the boil was cured and the draining wound had closed.

This demonstrates the use of increasing the blood to an area of trouble by utilizing moist heat. Such applications insure localization of the infectious process—keeping it confined to a small area and preventing spread of the infection. Increasing blood to the area increases white cells (these engulf bacteria and form what is commonly called pus) and antibodies to fight off the infection.
Such localized skin infections as Jack's do not need antibiotics as a general rule. Even if antibiotics are given, they can't get into the site of the infection since the white cells have formed a tight

ring around the infection preventing the entrance of the antibiotic into the "battle ground."

How to Get the Most from Your Temperature Thermostat

Another function of blood is as the body's sensitive heat regulator. Without it, no one can survive. When the body gets too hot the blood carries off the excess heat to the sweat glands where perspiration (sweating) gets rid of it. The blood also stimulates body cells to slow down their metabolism during hot spells, reducing that formation from metabolism until normal temperatures prevail.

Everyone has their own heat loss rate. If you've been sweating a lot, it means your body has been getting rid of heat from hard work or whatever. Getting rid of this heat takes salt—it's what the sweat glands use to radiate heat from your system.

HOW IRENE BEAT THE HEAT PROBLEM

I see a lot of cases like Irene F.'s. She came dragging into my office one day in midsummer complaining of ever increasing fatigue, mental dullness and weakness. She could barely move herself along and was obviously a sick lady.

In talking to Irene, I found that she'd been going through this every summer—always felt pretty good in winter. She hardly ever took salt in her diet, yet her work kept her busy, active and sweating all the time during summer months. She was depriving her blood of enough salt to get rid of her excess heat! And it was slowly making her an invalid.

Irene recovered almost immediately when she began to take salt tablets and extra fluids in the hot summer months and even in the winter if she perspired heavily doing whatever it was that made her work up a sweat. She gained back her strength, her pep, and energy and now leads a perfectly normal life.

HOW YOU CAN PROFIT FROM
BETTER BODY HEAT REGULATION

The main reason your body heat regulation is important is that there are certain tissues such as nerve cells that simply cannot tolerate too much elevated temperature above the normal 98.6 degrees Fahrenheit. The reproductive cells are other special cells that need constant temperature.

Barney C. is a good example of what happens when the blood loses control of its heat regulation control.

Barney started to work on a ranch in the high country during the summer. He wasn't used to the summer heat, having been a student during the rest of the year. He was brought into the hospital emergency room one hot summer day unconscious and in shock. When I saw Barney, his skin was warm, dry and seemed to lack the usual springiness when pinched—if I'd take a fold of skin between my thumb and first finger and elevate it, it would very slowly flatten out again instead of springing back to the flat position as it is supposed to do.

Barney's rectal temperature was 103 degrees Fahrenheit—about five degrees above normal. There was no sign of infection any-where. His blood pressure was low, and his pulse was rapid and felt "thready" instead of full and bounding as it usually does. Barney had neglected to compensate for his exertion for long hours in the hot sun at high altitude, and he'd suffered heat prostration or sun-stroke, as it's sometimes called.

HOW YOU CAN PREVENT SUNSTROKE
AND HEAT PROSTRATION

1. Always take in extra salt when doing physical exertion that makes you sweat. Even more extra salt should be added to this if you are working out of doors in the hot sun and in higher altitudes. Take three salt tablets a day for sweat work of normal variety; six if this is done in the hot sun; eight if at higher altitudes. Salt tablets should be taken *with meals* and with *ample fluids.*

2. You need to drink fluids every 30 to 45 minutes when working in hot weather and working up a sweat. Plain water will do, but any fluid is fine. You need anywhere from four to eight extra glasses of fluid over and above the usual ten or twelve glasses per day.

3. Any time you begin to feel sick—nausea and weakness—or have a headache when working in the sun, *stop,* seek shade and lie down. Take in fluids and salt when your stomach settles down.

4. Do not use plain table salt in very large quantities. It makes you nauseated especially if you use it on an empty stomach. Inexpensive commercial salt tablets are buffered and help prevent irritation of your stomach.

5. Rest frequently even if you feel well. There's nothing like preventing what Barney ended up with.

Barney responded to intravenous fluids and ice baths. He was "out of it" for about two weeks. He noticed that his tolerance to heat—how much he could exert in the sun—was definitely diminished following his heat stroke. This is usual for such reactions as Barney had to the heat. Give your blood a break— don't force it to do the impossible.

Better Blood Communications Functioning

Your blood carries vital messages to every cell, every fiber of your body. There are hundreds of such messages being carried along by your bloodstream each minute of your waking and sleeping life.

Hormones secreted by your endocrine glands are one type of message carried by your blood. Chemicals secreted by your liver and pancreas are another. Changes in various elements of your blood—blood sugar, fat levels, salt levels and so on—are yet others. You keep this messenger service at peak efficiency by continuous physical toning—yet another bonus from what you've accomplished by mastering Chapter 2. If you've been somewhat lax in getting your toning routines started, give your blood a break by starting them today!

Building a Better Nutrition Carrier Function

Consider this series of events:

1. You eat a meal. Food is broken down in the stomach and small intestine.
2. When digestion of food is completed in the intestine, basic elements of food—protein, carbohydrate and fats—are absorbed by special cells of the intestine.
3. When absorption has taken place, foodstuffs enter directly into tiny capillaries surrounding the intestine.
4. From capillaries, foodstuff is carried into bigger and bigger vessels where all of it enters the liver circulation for detoxification of any unwanted or unusable chemicals, and for storage of chemicals from which protein and other important elements are made.
5. From liver, blood carries *good stuff* to every cell in your body.

PHYSICAL TONING IMPROVES NUTRITION

When you stimulate your circulation—by exercise, for example, this process doubles or triples in speed and efficiency. Consider sit-ups, for example. Not only does this speed up circulation, but it also squeezes the liver every time you make your abdominal muscles pull you up off the floor to a sitting position. This forces fresh nutrients—proteins for building up spent muscle fibers, for example—into your blood to replace the hundreds of thousands of cells that wear out every hour in your body. It also speeds up the carrying of cell waste products back to the liver for elimination from your system. A double bonus as a result of your physical toning routines!

Your Body Depends on Its Waste Disposer

Still another of your blood's prime functions is the elimination of waste from your system. I've already described that carbon dioxide, the end point of cell metabolism, is exhaled by your lungs with each breath you take. The bloodstream carries this unusable product to your lungs for such elimination.

Your kidneys, the body's other major eliminator, have the richest blood supply of all your organs next to the lungs and liver. This is no coincidence—your entire blood volume is filtered through these remarkable organs in hundreds of miles of capillaries where the waste products are removed and forced into urine and eliminated.

Think how much this process is improved by physical toning. Think of toning routines as the way to stop all those wastes from piling up in your blood and cells. Start today getting out in that fresh air for an invigorating walk or going to the garage and hauling out that bicycle for transportation to run errands instead of the lazy way in a car. Start today getting your bloodstream humming with more flow for better health!

SUMMARY

1. Your blood is another of your body's tissues. The red and white cells and serum are special cells. Blood travels in vessels that react in proportion to how you keep your blood in health.

2. Your blood carries the keys to resistance to disease and temperature regulation. You can influence both these activities by practicing good principles of health.

3. Your blood is in touch with every cell, every fiber in your body, through hormone and chemical messengers. To keep these messages clear and on the track at all times, your blood must be stimulated by exercise and good nutrition.

4. Elimination of waste is a prime function of blood. If you let yourself become lazy and behave like a sloth, wastes will pile up. Start health control today to prevent this from happening.

5. To stay vital, your blood needs ample supplies of water and salt; more of both with hard physical labor at high altitudes in the sun.

5

How to Breathe Sparkling Health
into Your Lungs

Increased resistance, heart and blood vessels, and blood—these have been the targets of your journey toward health thus far. In this section, you'll see how you can deal with those important bellows inside your chest: your lungs.

You'll need to discover something, first of all, that most people don't know about, namely, how to breathe correctly. You'll also see how to look for and remove pollution from the air you breathe.

We'll take a look at the two major scourges of the human lungs—asthma and emphysema—and how to prevent and treat them both. Also covered will be the prevention and treatment of pneumonia and bronchitis—what causes them as well as the best way to prevent your voice box (larynx) from getting into trouble.

Finally, the problems of the correct way to treat your lungs during convalescence, and the problems of cancer and tuberculosis of the lungs are important. We'll look at both problems in this chapter.

HOW TO IMPROVE YOUR BREATHING

Most people don't know how to breathe properly. The reason is that they were never taught! Why this should be, I'm not sure, but proper breathing habits can and do make the difference between good health and poor health in far too many instances. Let's take a look at breathing technique for a minute.

Your chest is separated from your abdomen by two huge muscles, one on either side of your rib chest. The muscles are called the diaphragms. The diaphragms should be, but generally aren't, the *prime breathing muscles.*

On a chest X ray, you see both lung fields extending down to the diaphragms—the diaphragms appearing as dome-shaped, white shadows at the bottom of each lung. When you breathe in—inhale—these dome-shaped muscles flatten out, sucking in air. They flatten out, that is, *if you are using them to breathe.* If you're not using them to breathe, your chest cage expands to draw in the air, and in the long run this amounts to inefficient breathing! You need to *use* those muscles, the diaphragms.

Here Is the Way to Better Breathing

1. Sit in a chair, back straight. Now collapse your chest completely—blow all the air in your lungs out.
2. Now, take in a breath—*but don't allow your chest to expand.* You'll notice that your upper abdomen "pooches out" during this maneuver, if you're doing it properly. You'll also notice that you are taking in a lot of air and your chest hasn't even begun to expand as yet.
3. When you've sucked in all the air you can with your diaphragms, then allow your chest to expand, further filling your lungs with vital essential oxygen.

This is the proper way to breathe. With your diaphragms *and* your chest! There is no doubt about it, you can inhale about twice as much air with such improved breathing than if you breathe only with your chest!

How Dorothy Corrected Poor Breathing Habits

A middle-aged lady named Dorothy P. was having trouble with breathing during her toning routines. She was also having trouble with weight reduction. She couldn't, she said, seem to get enough air in during physical toning.

I asked Dorothy to breathe for me in the office. She was a chest breather—hardly used her diaphragms at all. After I taught Dorothy to breathe, not only did she do far better with exercises, but her weight problem seemed to be easier for her to handle—she lost weight more rapidly than before!

In Dorothy's case, I simply added an extra to her toning routines. She was to take ten deep breaths with her diaphragm *and* her chest before starting every exercise routine. She was to do this twice more during the middle of the day as well. Within a month, Dorothy was well on her road to health with better breathing, better weight control, and better physical toning.

HOW TO ELIMINATE INTERNAL POLLUTION

Your Program to Control Smoking

For the past ten to fifteen years, there has been a concerted effort on the part of many health authorities to eliminate smoking entirely from the American way of life. I've always felt their efforts to be too all-inclusive, but they are quite right in some respects.

My own view of smoking is that there are a few diseases and disorders in which smoking must be eliminated altogether. For the most part, however, *a reduction in amount is adequate to the purpose of reaching good health.* I'll mention the absolute *no smoking* situations as I go along in this chapter. The following is a list of things I consider just as harmful to health, if not more so, than smoking:

1. Alcoholism and overuse of drugs and medicine.
2. Environmental pollution.
3. Absence of physical toning routines.
4. Obesity.

As a general rule of thumb, *you should cut down your present smoking rate by 75 percent.* If you're smoking two packs of cigarettes a day, you can do quite well on 10 cigarettes a day. If you smoke one pack of cigarettes a day, you will bring your internal pollution to tolerable levels by cutting to 5 cigarettes a day.

One method to help cut down smoking is to switch to a pipe or to cigars as an alternate to cigarettes.

HOW SMOKING CAN BE TAMED BY USING ROD'S EXPERIENCE

Typical of hundreds of men I've known who have controlled this business of smoking is Rod, an inveterate smoker of 24 years, puffing away on two to three packs of cigarettes every day of the week. Rod's case was first called to my attention when he bitterly complained of short-windedness in physical toning sessions. He simply didn't have the breathing reserve to stick to his excercises.

Rod started to concentrate on the following suggestion just before slipping off to sleep at night: "Tomorrow, the taste of cigarettes will make me sick." Rod repeated this phrase several times, with nothing else cluttering his mind or diverting his attention. After several repetitions, Rod put the subject of smoking out of his mind completely. He forced his mind to think of something else entirely unrelated to smoking, then drifted off to sleep.

After three weeks of applying willpower, Rod could not tolerate smoking even one cigarette a day without becoming quite ill. He stopped completely. Rod hasn't smoked in three years and has regained his wind. He can jog four miles without tiring, and there is no calisthenic beyond his wind capacity.

Rod's case is not unusual, and it shows again how you have within you the capacity to do almost anything you decide to do!

HOW TO IMPROVE YOUR ENVIRONMENT

There are many hundreds of thousands of people today who go to work and breathe in unsafe air all the while they're earning a living. I'm not talking now about people who work in mines, rock quarries, foundries or chemical plants. These areas are well known for their production of ill health through lung pollution, and I'll not go into them at this time.

HOW HANK AND ALICE IMPROVED
THEIR WORKING ENVIRONMENT

I'm talking about people like Hank and Alice.

Hank:

Hank E. worked in a printing shop. He had been for seventeen years. About three years before I saw him, he began to develop shortness of breath and a dry, hacking cough. It was always after he got to work, and it always got better when he came home.

Extensive examination revealed no trouble as far as I could find. Eventually Hank was found to have a true allergy to printer's ink—or more accurately, one of the substances from which such ink is made. When he changed jobs, so as to avoid contact with the ink, his lungs cleared and his health has been excellent.

Alice:

Alice H. worked in the spotlessly clean, pure air environment of a pharmaceutical plant. She had been for ten years. She began to develop shortness of breath and chest pain on occasion, and noticed increasing numbers of respiratory infections every year. Her health was otherwise quite good and all tests proved nothing wrong.

Subsequent investigation of her work area revealed a fine, invisible powder in the air, hardly noticeable, especially to those who had worked there for some time. This dust was beginning to cause her lungs to react, not because of the chemical nature of the dust, just to its irritating physical presence in her lungs. Alice couldn't quit work, so she began to wear a mask for filtering out the dust while at work. All her symptons cleared and her lungs are healthy today.

CONTROLLING ALCOHOL FOR BETTER LUNGS

Although nothing much has been written about it, I've observed that chronic alcoholics have a high risk of having COPD—an abbreviation for chronic lung disease. Whether this is from the alcohol itself or from the poor nutrition that most alcoholics have, I don't know, and I don't think anybody else does. Suffice to say that, aside from all the other hazards of drinking too much alcohol, chronic, irreversible lung trouble can result.

I'll have more to say about alcoholism later in the book.

YOUR IMMEDIATE SURROUNDINGS ARE IMPORTANT

The following list of common mistakes that I find people make in their own homes will help you achieve lung health:

1. Even in the dead of winter, sleep with a source of fresh air coming into your bedroom. Your lungs—your entire body—constantly need fresh oxygen. The more you have to rebreathe stale musty air, the poorer your health will eventually become.

2. When you smell a gassy smell in your home, have it checked out by your utilities people. Both bottled and natural gas are odorless, but a chemical is usually added to it to make it smell if there should develop a leak to your furnace or hot water tank.

3. Always exercise with a fresh air source readily available to the room you're exercising in. Do as much outdoor exercising as you possibly can.

4. Make sure your furnace has a good ventilation system—have the furnace flue checked routinely every two or three years. The gas from a defective

furnace flue is *not* smellable! If you or any members of your household notice headaches only when at home, suspect trouble in your heating plant.

ENTIRE FAMILY SUFFERS FROM POOR HEATING SYSTEM

I vividly recall a situation in a small town in which I practiced where an entire family of six came home from the movies late one night and every one of them came down with nausea, vomiting, and headaches from a defective furnace flue that was spewing toxic carbon monoxide into the house.

Fortunately, no permanent ill effects resulted. But it could have been a catastrophe!

YOUR PROGRAM FOR PREVENTION AND TREATMENT OF EMPHYSEMA

Emphysema is of growing concern to medical people because they are seeing it with much more frequency these days. It's also true that more younger people are getting emphysema than ever before. Why is this? What is responsible? It isn't entirely settled, but certain things about it are very clear: *Emphysema, or a process similar to it, can arise in anyone's lungs from any irritant they inhale constantly over a period of time, coupled with continued poor habits of lung tone.*

With this in mind, I'll now come to the first exception to the smoking rule I discussed earlier in this chapter: *Not all people who smoke will get emphysema but almost 95 percent of all people who have emphysema either are or have been heavy smokers.*

HOW TO CONTROL YOUR IRRITATION TOLERANCE

In my opinion, every person has his own particular tolerance to irritating substances he may breathe in. For that matter, everyone has his particular tolerance to anything that may irritate any part of his body, such as sunlight, spicy foods, cosmetics or tight garters, for example.

In other words, every person has a limit to irritation and inflammation, past which he gets into trouble if the cause of the irritation continues. You can, for instance, smoke only so much—when you exceed this limit (your own unique tolerance), you have chest trouble. Some people can be out in the sun all the time and never seem to suffer. Others can burn and develop chronic skin disease with only an occasional exposure.

Emphysema is the same. It develops in one person with little in the way of exposure to irritants; in others only after long years of high exposure. And in still others, it never develops at all in spite of heavy, long continued exposure.

Emphysema is a chronic lung disorder in which the problem is difficulty in getting the breathed-in air *out of your chest.* It starts with shortness of breath while doing physical activity that never bothered one before. It may remain at this stage or progress (if something isn't done about it) to inability to breathe comfortably even at rest.

Your lungs are composed of millions of tiny air sacs—they resemble clusters of grapes under the microscope—that individually expand and contract with each breath you take. The muscle coat around the tiny sac is responsible for this movement.

In emphysema, these tiny air sacs expand alright, but they lose their ability to contract. Air is trapped inside the millions of tiny air sacs. Neither carbon dioxide nor oxygen can be exchanged as usual under such conditions. Air hunger results.

The Following Rules Will Be Helpful to You in Preventing Emphysema

1. Keep your smoking at an absolute minimum (5 cigarettes a day or less).
2. Avoid occupations where irritating fumes or dust are a problem.
3. Start physical toning and proper breathing *today.*
4. If you have allergies that involve your lungs, take steps to have them cleared up.

HOW YOU CAN PROFIT FROM JIM'S EXPERIENCE IN COMBATING EMPHYSEMA

Jim P., a Rocky Mountain rancher, had developed emphysema before I had him as a patient. When I first saw him, he was 48 years old, had noted shortness of breath on exertion for about a year, and had difficulty throwing off chest colds. He usually ended up on antibiotics with each cold he'd had for the past year.

Jim's Anti-Emphysema Routine

1. The "balloon" exercise at least four times a day. I instructed Jim to go to the dime store and pick up a package of thick-skinned kid's balloons and to keep a fresh supply on hand all the time. Four times a day, I had Jim

simply blow up a balloon, then let the air out again. He was to repeat this for two or three minutes at first, gradually building up the time he spent blowing until he was doing at least ten minutes worth.

2. I started Jim on physical toning routines. He couldn't handle much more than some of the less strenuous isometrics at first. However, within six weeks, Jim progressed to some calisthenics and in twelve weeks to some jogging.

3. Jim had been an inveterate smoker for 26 years. I made him stop completely. He did this by first switching to a pipe while he cut down his cigarettes. He stopped smoking completely inside two months.

4. Diaphragm breathing. Jim practiced this at least three times a day for ten to fifteen minutes.

5. Within three months, I asked Jim to enroll at a local YMCA and start swimming lessons. He just about gave up the whole routine, he got so tired, but persistence paid off. Within another six months, Jim could swim three pool lengths.without resting.

Jim was fortunate. He was able to eradicate his emphysema symptons in about a year's time. He hasn't had it back, and won't as long as he keeps himself in good health.

HOW TO DEAL WITH ASTHMA

The "big three" causes of asthma are: allergy; infection; emotion. Some asthma involves a combination of two or more of them, but often pure cases are caused, for example, by an allergic reaction to weeds, flowers, molds, trees, grasses and the like.

How Ilene Controlled Her Allergies

Ilene B. is a good example of someone with primarily allergic type asthma. Since she could recall, Ilene had itchy eyes, sneezing, and coughing in the spring and fall of the year with the coming into bloom and pollination of a variety of growing things. By the time Ilene became a teenager, she was beginning to have the wheeze so characteristic of asthma in addition to her nose, throat and eye problems. Testing revealed few, if any, types of plant life that she wasn't allergic to.

During the spring and fall of the year, Ilene could bring on an attack of asthma simply by physical exertion. When I saw Ilene the first time, she was on three different medicines, and needed another to make her wheezing tolerable.

Ilene was able to completely control her asthma by first being thoroughly desensitized to the pollens she was allergic to. This took about three years to accomplish, but if you could see Ilene today, enjoying swimming, skiing, cycling and any other activity she wishes without asthma, you would agree that it was worth the time.

Today, Ilene doesn't have to use any medicines. She has done well on physical toning routines. I'm certain these had as much to do with her cure as the desensitizing, but with so much to deal with, her pollen shots were the the only sensible way to start. Desensitizing involves simply taking injections in quite dilute amounts of the things you are sensitive to. This is determined by skin tests. After a time, your body builds up a resistance to these sensitizers, so that breathing in pollen from them no longer trips off the allergic or asthmatic response.

How Carl Threw Off Recurrent Infection Shackles

Carl G. had asthma from reaction to infections. He was free of asthma except when he had a cold, a chest infection, or an infected tooth. At these times, he'd wheeze like an old steam engine. When the infection cleared up, Carl wouldn't have asthma any more.

To deal with Carl's case, I started him on health control. Within a year's time, Carl had progressed with physical toning and resistance building so well that his resistance to cold, flu, and other infections was ironclad. He simply didn't have infections any longer. And with the infections and colds went the asthma. He hasn't been troubled since!

How Joanne Triumphed Over the Emotional Basis for Her Asthma.

Of all the causes of asthma, emotional distress is, in my opinion, the most common. It's also the hardest to deal with since many people unconsciously use their wheezing attacks (they can be so severe as to turn the patient blue at times) to control the people with whom they come in contact—use their asthma to manipulate their surroundings, so to speak.

Joanne was such a patient. Joanne was on four different medicines for her asthma when I first met her. She would go from a week to six months without an attack, then have one attack of wheezing after another for several days running. When I learned that Joanne's trouble was from purely emotional causes she and I began to work toward her asthma control.

The first thing I did was to find out why she needed to control things by wheezing. It didn't take long to find out that it was a direct reaction to the rigid, demanding, completely inflexible way in which Joanne's parents raised her. She was rebelling in the only way she knew how—with repeated attacks of asthma when the going got tough.

First of all, I persuaded Joanne's parents to let up. To let her move in with an aunt who lived nearby, and to stay out of Joanne's life entirely. This was difficult, but they finally agreed. Next, I began the ground work for health control. The physical toning was easy since Joanne was young, lithe and in good shape anyway. It was the emotional control that was difficult.

Eventually, Joanne gained insight into her problem by accepting the reasons for her asthma attacks. Still they came on. Then she learned she could stop them cold when she felt them coming on by lying down and concentrating on the phrase, "My breathing tubes and air sacs will expand," over and over again, then putting any thought of herself or her asthma out of her mind completely. (Asthma is just the opposite of emphysema. The little air sacs contract down in spasm instead of expanding—air is hard to get *in* in contrast to emphysema where it's hard to get *out*.)

In three months, Joanne was able to get more involved with physical exertion without provoking an attack. Finally, she succeeded in preventing 75 percent of her asthma attacks. When she feels one coming on, she is able to stop about three in four of them—quite a record considering how disabled she was before mastering health control.

HOW TO MANAGE PNEUMONIA, BRONCHITIS AND PLEURISY

How to Recognize Pneumonia

Pneumonia is an infectious process that involves lung tissues. Many more cases of pneumonia are diagnosed every winter than actually are pneumonia because it has become a favorite disease to have. Besides this, it's easier to get people to take antibiotics with pneumonia than with just bronchitis, which most pneumonia cases turn out to be.

True pneumonia will generally present the following symptoms. If they're not there, it probably isn't pneumonia:

1. Temperature above 102 degrees. Chills, aching and feeling very sick generally.

2. Cough—phlegm, usually greenish or blood tinged. Feeling of painful fullness in chest.

3. Breathing is difficult, painful, rapid and labored. When penumonia really occurs, it should be treated in a hospital. Much more common is:

How to Get On Top of Bronchitis:

1. Temperature varies from normal to 101 degrees. Aching, but can get around.

2. Cough—some phlegm, often dry and hacky. Midline burning discomfort in chest.

3. Breathing may be uncomfortable, but not labored or rapid.

The following rules will help you successfully handle most bronchitis:

1. Stay indoors; no open windows at night; plenty of rest.

2. Use aspirin freely—two tablets every three or four hours.

3. Warm moist packs over congested area of chest after thorough rub with oil of wintergreen solution.

COLD PILLS OFTEN HINDER

Cold capsules and pills all contain drugs called antihistamines which are to dry up runny noses. This is all well and good but the breathing tubes in your lungs are irritated and dry anyway—these pills and capsules usually make matters worse if bronchitis is present. They're better avoided.

HOW TO TREAT HOARSENESS

With flu and colds and a host of other respiratory trouble in the fall, winter and spring or even in mild weather, the problem of "croakiness" comes up. When you get hoarse—sometimes lose your voice entirely—you have laryngitis.

Your voice feels and sounds as though it's coming out of a barrel.

YOUR BEST ROUTINE FOR LARYNGITIS

1. Stop smoking and stop talking! That's right—no using the voice. Just

whisper or write down your messages. After all, your vocal cords are irritated. They need rest.

2. Avoid the night air. No night air through the windows during sleep. Cold air is very irritating to inflamed vocal cords.

3. Add two or three tablespoons of Compound Tincture of Benzoin (available without a prescription from the drug store) in two or three inches of water in a sauce pan or old skillet. Heat this mixture on the stove on a medium burner setting and inhale the fumes in through your mouth as they rise from the pan. The fumes must pass directly over your strained and ailing vocal cords during this maneuver. Repeat this as many times as you wish during the day and evening. Pills and lozenges that you suck in your mouth can't reach the spots of trouble.

If any hoarseness fails to yield to this method in a week's time, always, ALWAYS let your doctor take a look at your vocal cords with a small throat mirror used for this purpose.

HOW TO MAINTAIN HEALTHY LUNGS WHILE CONVALESCING

If for any reason you must be in bed or must convalesce by resting at home, recall that you can keep your lungs—and therefore you blood, heart and body cells—in reasonably good condition by practicing deep breathing (ten forced breaths in and ten forced breaths out) followed by three or four coughs several times a day. You can do this even when flat in bed, though it can be made a little easier by propping your chest and head up a little.

HOW TO DETECT TUBERCULOSIS AND CANCER

Fortunately, tuberculosis is declining greatly as a dread disease in this country. It still occurs, but not often. If it should occur (and if you're practicing good principles of lung health discussed in this chapter, it probably won't) face it with strong heart—it can be cured.

Tuberculosis Danger Signs

1. Weight loss; cough that doesn't clear up; and night sweats.
2. Change in personality (irritability); severe fatigue out of line with physical activity; and shortness of breath.

Cancer of the lungs is on the upswing in this country. There are people who claim lung cancer is preventable—all you need to do is stop smoking, or better, never start. The fact is that although it can't be prevented entirely, it can undoubtedly be cut down a great deal by curbing your smoking.

MY ADVICE ABOUT LUNG CARE

1. After 40 years of age, drastically reduce smoking or completely switch from cigarettes to pipe or cigars.

2. If there is any suggestion of lung cancer in your family tree (parents, grandparents, uncles, aunts) stop smoking altogether, preferably before the age of 35. Seek a nonirritating environment to work in. Avoid working around chemicals, dust, smoke, irritating gasses, and the like.

3. Practice diligently the principles of health as given in this book. Do not let up; do not give up; do not be misled—*there is no substitute for following good health principles and having yearly checkups by your medical advisor in fighting off and preventing most forms of cancer!*

4. Chest X rays are the most useful tools we have for picking up early lung diseases. Get a chest X ray every two or three years.

SUMMARY

1. Breathing correctly tones lungs and helps avoid internal pollution. You should practice it daily.

2. Both emphysema and asthma are potential cripplers. Both can be prevented and both can be cured. Don't let either handicap your chances for lasting health.

3. Good resistance to pneumonia, bronchitis, and laryngitis can be had by attention to health control. All three are treatable and if present, need not halt your progress to health.

4. Tuberculosis is declining, but still can be a threat to health. It can be treated. Cancer of the lungs can be minimized by common sense—cured if discovered early. Periodic checkups by your medical specialist usually includes chest X rays—the most important tool in the discovery of tuberculosis and cancer.

6

How to Put a Solid Punch into
Your Nervous System

Of all the tissues of your body. Your nerves take the worst beating day in and day out. When you consider the fact that nerves are the first to receive the thousands of sensations from your every day world, and that they transmit, integrate, and then send back action messages to every organ and muscle in your body, it's no wonder they take the brunt of the stresses and strains of life! In this section you'll discover how to protect your nerves and how to make them work at top efficiency all the time.

Your nerves have certain capacities that few people take time to learn about. You should know what these potentials are, how you use them, and what to do when they're out of whack.

Any discussion of nerves must also involve the care and feeding of your brain—the seat of your most valuable possession, your mind. We'll look at the brain and its care in this chapter.

Living with nerves, that is, learning to control them so you may remain in top physical health, is important. You'll learn ways and means of insuring dynamic nerve health.

HOW TO AVOID WEAR AND TEAR ON YOUR NERVES

The art of knowing how and when to relax is rapidly becoming lost. I confess I have little sympathy with patients who come to me looking and feeling frazzled and worn out, saying "I just can't keep up with my job," or "My family is just getting me down," and then asking for something to stimulate them during the day and something else to put them to sleep at night.

It's all so unnecessary! It's also a waste of human tissue and health.

Three Steps to Complete Relaxation

1. Get your body into a position such that *all* your muscles can go limp. You can be sitting with your legs propped up or reclining or lying down.

2. Put all thought of current business and/or problems out of your mind completely—close your eyes if you want to. Gaze into space with your eyes open, but get your mind on something far away from the business at hand.

3. Concentrate on your muscle groups one at a time; concentrate and silently repeat the phrase, "My muscles will relax and get soft" several times.

It's amazing what just doing these three steps once or twice during the day can do for your nerves. I know it sounds simple—almost ridiculous, but I suggest you may not really understand what relaxation is if you haven't tried it. I further suggest you try it before you knock it. Just make it a point to do the routine twice a day for a week or two. I'll wager you'll increase your efficiency and feel so much better once you get used to it that you'll make it a part of your daily habit.

HOW TO TAKE A GENUINE "BREAK"

Many people are under the impression that the two or more coffee breaks they take every working day is for relaxation. Actually, most people do anything but relax—they swill black coffee and engage in constant chatter with someone else. This can make you more unstrung than before the break.

1. Better than coffee is skim milk. Coffee is a good pick-me-up but should be taken with either an artificial creamer (the powdered kind—it's defatted) or something to eat. This is to prevent your blood sugar from taking a dive as a result of the caffeine in coffee. Low blood sugar produces shakiness, hunger pangs, feelings of panic (blue mood), jitteriness, and restlessness. It may even make you upset and impair your judgment—hardly the kind of things you want from a break.

2. Make it a point to exercise. Stir up that circulation; flex as many muscles as you can; breathe deeply of fresh air. In other words, get away from the environment and practice the good principles of health control you've already learned.

3. Follow this with the three steps to complete relaxation I mentioned previously.

How to Practice Meditation

With relaxation and the break, the art of meditation follows naturally. How long has it been since you really meditated? When you meditate, you dwell deeply in your thoughts while completely relaxed—you muse, you think. And such thoughts are about the things in your life that are really important. Not your job; not your next raise or the guy that's running the office. Rather, the loved ones in your family; your direction in life; the important social issues of the day or whether you're profiting by past mistakes—these are the things worth meditating about.

Meditation was practiced by the ancients and is practiced by certain religions and creeds today. What are they really doing? Is something magical happening? Are meditations mystical and not open to the general public?

Meditations are used today just as they were used in ancient times-for relaxation to a depth not reached in most situations; for getting yourself together; for arriving, if you will, at *total health control!*

Real meditation is best done in surroundings conducive to deep relaxation and concentration. Home is the natural setting. It isn't necessary to meditate more than once or twice a week, but meditation will help you see yourself in different lights and help you arrive at dynamic health more quickly and stay with it over the long haul.

1. Assume the elements for relaxation listed earlier in this chapter.
2. Now form a picture in your mind's eye of whom or what you want to meditate about—one of your children, for example, or yourself, if this is what you want to consider.
3. Let no other thoughts enter your mind except this picture. Concentrate on the face or the object to the exclusion of all else. Now begin to let your mind take over. Let it roam, swing, rove and analyze, but always with the picture of the object or person first and foremost in your mind's eye.

How Venting Brings on Peace of Mind

Venting means letting off steam when the pressure's on. It's a way to get rid of unwanted, unhealthful pressure, anger, frustration and the like, and to prevent your nervous system from having to take the brunt of an emotional build-up. Venting also prevents your mind from having to play tricks on your body in channeling such build-ups over pathways that end up giving you heartburn, belly cramps, or palpitations. In Chapter 3, Betty is an example of such channeling.

There are different ways of venting as described below:

1. Clark P. was a loner type—quiet, firm in his ways and with a tendency to keep things bottled up. He could tell when he needed venting because he began to have a particular person or event turning over and over in his mind for hours or even for a day or two after whatever or whoever caused Clark to be upset. He was, in other words, ruminating—mentally chewing on his emotions. When this happened, Clark found that sudden bursts of calisthenics—a half hour spent punching a stuffed pillow he had at home—got rid of the trouble. His venting was characterized by a controlled, *explosion* activity of some kind.

2. Judy N. was good natured, affable and outgoing. She never hesitated to tell others what she thought or to tell off any one who needed it. Still, Judy could feel pressure building inside, especially during situations where people indicated she could do a better job or hinted she wasn't doing something right.

Judy found the best way to vent such a build-up was to get involved with something that took her mind completely off the situation. She was an expert with knitting needles, and found 45-60 minutes spent knitting vented such feeling satisfactorily. And the bonus was there in extra sweaters and afghans she wouldn't have made otherwise.

3. Tim A. worked in a factory full of people. When he became worked up about something or someone, his best vent, he found, was to immediately "blow his stack." Tim found if he didn't, he'd develop all kinds of physical symptoms all day long and for a day or two afterward. He was on his way to having a stomach ulcer before he started his venting.

Tim didn't get violent or out of control, but his employees knew that when he *blew* somebody had goofed—they heard about it, and then it was done. No grudges, no afterburning, no marks on the record—and everybody was happy.

HOW TO MASTER THE ART OF RELIEVING PAIN

Pain has always been mankind's greatest enigma. It's difficult to deal with because pain means something different for each person who has it. It's usually a matter of intensity, and how you're conditioned to deal with it.

As a general rule, pain is your body's way of telling you that something is wrong. It doesn't mean that the wrong area is in danger necessarily, but rather that normal function has been interrupted. Types and varieties of pain run the gamut from the *sharp* pin-prick to the throbbing *migraine headache.* From the continuous searing pain caused by burns to the deep aching pain caused by a twisted ankle. Regardless of the cause, pain demands relief even though your nerves may be playing tricks and making you think more pain is there than is actually the case.

How to Control Injury Pains

Ever notice how a muscle in good shape is far less susceptible to pain from injury than one that is soft and flabby? It's true. This is another reason why athletes want to keep in shape—the more solid and physically toned their muscles are, the more pounding, twisting, bruising and wrenching their muscles can take without hurting.

A simple rule of thumb about injuries is: If you put the injured part properly at rest, most of the pain should go away. The same with a broken bone: If properly set, the deep intense pain stops.

THE BEST AGENTS TO USE FOR INJURY PAIN

1. The first 48 hours: Application of cold—ice packs are the best way to accomplish this. Ice injured areas for 30 minutes four times daily.
2. The next period (after 48 hours): application of heat—hot moist packs; a hot water bottle; heating pads and the like. *Note:* Don't burn the skin in your effort to apply heat, but keep the heat high and constant.
3. In strained or sprained ankles, knees, or any other joints: If weight bearing in normal use is painful, don't force it. Put the injured part at rest. If a leg is involved, get off it entirely or use crutches; if an arm is involved, put it in a sling (stuffing your hand and forearm inside your shirt or blouse may be enough).

How You Can Help Injured Joints

Any joint that has been injured and swells is going to do better under any circumstances if it's given support—so that when you do go about your activities, the joint doesn't wobble around. You can use adhesive tape, elastic wraps or almost anything to stabilize a joint. Before any adhesive material is applied to skin, you should paint the entire skin area well with compound tincture of benzoin and allow to dry. The application of plain talcum powder liberally on your skin will protect it from damage from perspiration while it's covered.

How to Deal with Headache Pain

Headache is perhaps the most common affliction of modern

man. Fortunately, headaches are usually harmless and don't mean a catastrophe is about to happen. The following table will help you decide whether your headache is serious or not:

Non Serious	Serious
Starts in the back of neck	Starts deep inside the head.
May feel like a band around head.	Severe pain—mostly in front.
Comes on during course of day.	Awakened from sleep with it.
May feel sick, but no vomiting.	Vomiting follows head pains.
State of consciousness not affected.	Black-outs, vision difficulties.

HOW TO MANAGE THE MOST COMMON TYPE OF HEADACHE

The most common form of headache is the headache caused from tension—from nerves being mangled; from being on edge; from being under too much pressure or overly fatigued. It generally starts in the neck and may work up to involve the sides and front of your head. It may be continuous pain or throbbing. Ida's method of dealing with such headaches was efficient, safe and certain. And it required no harsh drugs.

How to Use Ida's Plan for Your Tension Headache

Ida was 35, married and was busy with children; busy with housework; busy with community work in her prairie state village. In other words, Ida was probably too busy for her own good. However, she was serious about everything she did and she did not want to give any of it up just because of her headaches. But she was at a point where something had to give. If it didn't, Ida would have to start taking stronger drugs to control the pain which had become incapacitating at times.

When she first felt a tension headache coming on, Ida found that a special routine stopped them. Eventually, she was able to control them so well that they became only minor irritations. They happened less and less frequently and Ida will probably be able to stop them completely in due time.

The step Ida found helpful at the very first sign of tightness in the back of her head was to rub oil of wintergreen into her neck. She followed this by the application of heat—either a hot water bottle or hot moist packs using wash cloths soaked in simmering hot water on the stove. As one pack would cool down, another one, soaking in the simmering water, was used to replace it while the cooled cloth went back into the hot water. She kept this up for ten or fifteen minutes. When she felt her tight neck muscles relaxing, she took three aspirin and found someplace to lie flat on her back. She closed her eyes and concentrated on the phrase: "My neck muscles will relax." She repeated this phrase over and over again, and at the same time relaxed her entire body as well.

At first, Ida found herself drifting off into sleep, so good was her power of concentration. In about two months, she was able to avoid having to sleep to banish her headaches—she could stop them in about five minutes.

Today, Ida can simply concentrate, in any position, for two or three minutes and without the heat packs or aspirin, she can completely abort her tension headache.

The following table will help you to concentrate on the appropriate areas in different kinds of pain:

Type of Pain	Concentration Areas
Tension headaches.	Muscles in neck tight: Need to relax.
Migraine headaches.	Blood vessels dilated. Need to constrict.
Sinus headache.	Capillaries dilated (membranes congested) Need to constrict.
Injuries with swelling.	Capillaries dilated: Need to constrict (this removes the swelling from serum that gathers around wound).

HOW TO GET CONTROL OF NERVES THAT CAUSE THE MAJORITY OF PAINS

Yes, it's true, nerves are the seat for fully 60 percent of all the common ills that beset human beings. It seems that with our control of plagues, pestilence, famine and so forth—the scourges of ancient times—we have dealt ourselves into a position where nerves are the most vulnerable tissues of our bodies.

It's usually much simpler than you might suspect to interrupt patterns in your life that bring out the worst in your nerves. It takes a little self analysis as to what the *real* trouble is. Often the obvious escapes us. We live too close to it.

PROFIT FROM JAKE'S EXPERIENCE

You may, for example, find yourself in somewhat the same position as Jake R., a man I saw complaining of chronic pain in his lower back. There had been no injuries, no occupational changes, and nothing was found on examination or X ray to account for Jake's pain. Sometime later, I found out during a conversation with him that his pain developed at about the same time that his mother-in-law moved into their home for a prolonged visit. Frankly, Jake admitted, she gave him a pain in his—backside. She was always critical; always discontented; always arguing with Jake's decisions.

It wasn't until his mother-in-law left the home some time later that Jake got rid of the nagging pain in his backside. Yes, you can develop pain in any area the situation seems to dictate. Jake really had a pain in his backside because that's precisely where his mother-in-law made it settle!

MILLY LEARNS TO HANDLE DEBILITATING FACE PAIN

You could find your situation similar to Milly H.'s case. Milly had an affliction that is really a problem to handle—she had cluster face pain—sometimes called *tic douloureux*. This type of face discomfort is indeed painful, often requiring narcotic drugs to control. Fortunately, the disease is not common, and is most often seen in women—a fact that's not coincidental. There are more nervous women than men—it's just the way they're built.

At any rate, Milly was a typically hysterical person—she was nervous, quick to take up a cause, an argument or an underdog's side. None of these things by themselves of course, make one hysterical unless he lets it. Milly had. And the result was face pain of such severe nature that when I first saw her, she was asking for codeine, a narcotic drug, to control her pain.

How Milly Controlled Her Nerves

I decided to have a long talk about health with Milly, and I finally convinced her to try it. Within a year, Milly was able to control her hysteria—her extreme anxiety—by controlling her nerves. When this bridge was crossed, she was able to handle the face pain by lying flat in bed or on a couch and concentrating on the phrase: "The main nerve on the right side of my face is becoming numb." She repeated this several times, then pushed all thoughts of pain and nerves from her mind completely.

Today, Milly isn't absolutely free from *tic douloureux,* but she can stop a severe attack within minutes of its onset, and doesn't use anything stronger than aspirin!

How Fred Relieved His Tight Nerves

You may also profit from Fred T.'s case. Fred was a rancher and very active in Grange and Cattlemen's Association work in his community. Without previous trouble, Fred started developing chest pain on the left side—chest pain he immediately thought might be heart trouble. But in examining Fred I found no evidence of heart or lung trouble, nor for that matter any other trouble with his health.

Fred's trouble started when a new Cattlemen's Association president took office. From what I gathered, the new president was a vindictive, quarrelsome man who brooked no opinions other than his own and who ran things with *an iron fist*. Whenever Fred went to a meeting where this man was present, he had an attack later on.

When I presented Fred with the facts and could assure him that his physical health was perfect, he began to accept what (or whom) was the cause of his trouble. But what to do about it? He settled on direct confrontation. During a meeting, he summoned up his courage (Fred was rather shy and quiet), stood up and told the president he was dead wrong. When the man replied something to the effect that he thought Fred was out of order, Fred called him an "overbearing ass." The meeting broke up and Fred was backed unanimously by the rest of the members.

Fred has conditioned himself to stand up to people more—to speak out when he feels they're wrong. He has had no more chest pain.

HOW LOW BLOOD SUGAR CONTROL HELPS YOUR NERVES

Ever develop what I call the mid morning or mid afternoon blood sugar blues? This is when you suddenly feel jittery, jumpy, on edge, and weak. Ever go through a rough day at work, eating too much at mealtime and belting down more than your share of black coffee, only to arrive home with a ravenous appetite? Ever eat far too much after a couple of slugs of booze, then lapse into a stupor for the rest of the evening?

If this sounds familiar, it should. I estimate about 40 or 50 million people go through one or more of these low blood sugar blues episodes each day, and this may be a conservative estimate!

For a more complete discussion of low blood sugar and how to correct it, please refer to my book, *Low Blood Sugar, A Doctor's Guide to Its Effective Control,* Parker Publishing Company, 1969. Meantime, the following useful guides will help you to keep your blood sugar at proper levels and help your nerves hum with energy.

YOUR PROGRAM TO CONTROL LOW BLOOD SUGAR

1. Eat more sensibly. All of us would be better off if we adopted the Scandinavian habit of eating six smaller meals a day. At least plan to take a snack at mid morning, mid afternoon and in the evening. It shouldn't be a full course meal, just a snack with more protein content than carbohydrate. (*For example:* Two double soda crackers with peanut butter and a slab of American cheese between them).

2. Use coffee sensibly. Limit your intake to four cups a day. If you drink it black, never drink it without a snack. Use one of the powdered creamers if you wish, or skimmed milk, but don't drink it black on an empty stomach.

3. Review Chapters 1 and 2. Keep at them until you have reached the stage where your endocrine glands are in working harmony with your brain and nervous system.

4. Reduce alcohol consumption by 75 percent today. A glass or two of Sherry wine taken before supper or following your evening toning routine will do more for your nervous system than all the sedatives and tranquilizers ever made.

5. Plan to take in much more fruit juices and fresh fruits than before. The sugar in fruits doesn't go through the usual insulin cycle in your body's metabolism and is far more efficient in correcting low blood sugar than the sweets you usually eat, such as doughnuts, pie, cake, and sweet rolls.

A GUIDE TO THE CARE AND FEEDING OF YOUR BRAIN

Every nerve in your body has its origin in your brain. Your brain is by far the most efficient switchboard in existence today—all the fancy computers and the claims made for them notwithstanding! In addition to this, your brain is the seat of your mind—the thinking, creating, decision making, planning and emotional center. And your brain does all these things on less power than it takes to operate a single ordinary Christmas tree light bulb!

Your brain needs two things constantly and in high concentration: oxygen and sugar. Proper diet and breathing are essential to get proper levels of these two vital ingredients.

How to Increase Your Awareness

I'm amazed at the number of people I talk to every day who have allowed their brains to become fallow—let their minds get lazy, in other words. You can keep your brain tuned up for any challenge by just making it work. Does this take genius? Does it require a vast educational background? The answer to both questions is no. It takes only desire on your part.

Consider what you've already learned about the mind: that it can solve problems; that it can create; that it may have capacities that are untapped by most of us. Such an exceptional piece of mechanism needs tuning up once in a while. You can start your tuning as a patient of mine did.

LEE ANNE'S AWARENESS ADVENTURE

Lee Anne O. was a young lady in her 30's. She was married, had a family, and for all intent and purpose seemed happy and well adjusted. One day I was talking with Lee Anne about one of a succession of vague, ill-defined complaints having no basis in physical illness. Lee Anne admitted, as she put it, "I don't know, Doctor, I just seem to be sinking deeper and deeper into a rut that I can't climb out of." This, of course, was what was giving rise to all the vague aches and distresses.

In talking with Lee Anne further, I found that there had been nothing to challenge her, nothing to put her mind to work on solving problems—her husband having taken over all the duties of running the house, the finances and everything else. In fact, Lee Anne's life was being ground out, without anyone meaning it to, like a robot. Each day seemed more and more of a drudge to Lee Anne. There was nothing in her life that kept Lee Anne's brain *aware*. This had finally come to the stage where if something did pop up to challenge Lee Anne a little, she probably wouldn't recognize it or be able to act on it.

Awaken Your Brain

Lee Anne awakened her brain and her nerves by observing the following routine:

1. She started physical toning. We talked about mental toning as well. She

was skeptical, but finally agreed to try one thing. Each night after physical toning, she was to lie down in bed and concentrate on the phrase: "When I awaken in the morning, I'll feel relaxed, well, and eager to start a project." We left the project up in the air—I felt certain Lee Anne's mind would come up with what for her would prove the most interesting.

2. When I saw her next, she had decided to do something she'd held in the back of her mind for many years before she was married—she decided to take up writing.

3. With the decision made, Lee Anne's life seemed to change completely. She became brighter, more cheerful and looked forward to the challenge with great zest.

4. I advised Lee Anne to first of all, join a local writers' club. Not a professional organization, but a writer's club composed of others just like herself—amateurs with a desire to improve their writing. She did this, as well as making a trip to the library to check out several very good books on writing technique, publisher's needs and what they'll read and won't read, and some others.

Enjoy the Same Benefits Lee Anne Found!

I've seldom seen such a change in a patient. No longer was she dreading each passing day. No longer was there that dull look in her face—the lackluster expression that characterizes someone who is on the brink of a severe depression. She tackled the writing project with a vengeance. And meanwhile, she became a real mother to her children and a stimulating and interesting wife to her husband, who incidentally was quite skeptical at first about his wife's new pet interest.

Lee Anne reached health for the first time in many a moon. To date she has published six short stories and is working on a book length novel. Not bad for someone who was about to give up on everything!

Look Closely Around You

The point is, there is always something around—usually close at hand—that can stimulate you, make you aware of something you weren't aware of before, make you interested in doing something about it. In Lee Anne's case, that something was a long-buried yearning to write. It might be an interest in someone; a group less fortunate than yourself; a long forgotten interest in a field of study; a hobby; an avocation. Whatever it may be, you can resurrect it by using Lee Anne's technique.

HOW TO PREVENT ALCOHOL FROM DULLING YOUR BRAIN

In my work at a mental hospital these past five years, I've seen many great tragedies of the human condition. One of the worst, it seems to me, is the mental deterioration taking place in chronic alcoholics—the real alcoholics who have been in and out of such treatment centers for years.

Alcohol is quite capable of destroying your most prized possession—your brain, and with it your mind. Usually before this happens, however, comes deterioration of one or more nerves.

The Beginning of the End

Every day I see patients who can't move their left leg too well anymore or have lost the feeling in their right hand or who have no ability to tell when their rectums or bladders are full and are in a continual mess from the uncontrolled emptying of both these organs.

Of course there is good reason for their plights. They have, in their alcoholic excesses, allowed their nutrition to "go to pot." There is also a direct effect on nerve cells from alcohol, over a long period of time, that makes them degenerate.

Vitamin B Can Help You

I've already given you the rule of thumb about alcohol; about cutting down; about converting to wine in medium amounts at the proper time for efficient relaxation. This kind of alcohol intake never harmed anyone that I'm aware of. I have one thing for you to remember, however, if you feel your alcohol intake is more than it should be and are having difficulty cutting it down.

Make it a point to take in rather large quantities of Vitamin B complex, especially Thiamine (Vitamin B_1). If anything will help prevent nerve damage in the face of large alcohol intake, the B vitamins will. The dose of B complex is four tablets or capsules daily, and for thiamine it is at least 100 milligrams daily.

HOW TO LIVE WITH YOUR NERVES

The following program will help you with various nerve problems:

1. If you have epilepsy, you need to be on medicine to control the

seizures. The more they are out of control, the more chance for brain and nerve damage.

2. If you have already had a head injury of any kind, you need to work extra hard to prevent another. You should strive to look for situations (horseback and motor cycle riding, for example) that carry with them high risks of head injury and avoid them completely.

3. If you use alcohol excessively and notice signs of nerve control trouble, you must use the elements of good health and lots of vitamin B. At the same time, you must begin to cut your alcohol intake.

4. The way to break a mood—a period where you know you're in a rut because of anger, depression or whatever—is to get involved with something completely apart from your usual interests. Throw yourself into it. Get involved wholeheartedly, eagerly and without reservation. Such nerve moods will usually pass automatically.

SUMMARY

1. It's important to your health that you know how and when to relax; how and when to vent (let off steam). Practice can make you adept at these vital maneuvers.

2. Nerves are the basis for the majority of all ills. If not the basis, they can make any disorder seem much worse. One way to alleviate *nerves* is by learning to control pain.

3. Your brain and nerves depend on essential oxygen and sugar in plentiful amounts at all times. Low blood sugar blues may be damaging to your nerves. You can control low blood sugar easily and permanently.

4. Alcohol abuse and other nerve damaging situations all ultimately depend for their cure on practices of health control. Damaging effects on nerves may be reversed or halted by practicing these principles and by taking in extra Vitamin B Complex, especially Thiamine.

7

How to Build Lasting
Kidney and Bladder Health

Your kidneys and bladder are the first line of defense against the pile-up of waste products in your system. You will learn how to take care of these vital organs in this chapter. Infections in the urinary tract are not uncommon and you will also find out how to improve your capacity to prevent them and what to do if they occur.

Kidney and bladder function will serve you well if these organs are properly cared for. Nature has provided for this function to be continuous and sustaining, by her amazing structure of these organs. You will find and utilize the basic facts concerning their structure and function in this section. Kidney stones can become a problem. You should know what to do to stave off this uncomfortable condition.

No discussion of the urinary tract could be complete without talking about troubles occurring in the male prostate and the female uterus and cervix. Both of these will be considered in this chapter. Finally, the problem of venereal disease (VD) is important since such diseases invade your system through the urinary tract. VD will come under consideration in this chapter.

HOW TO PREVENT URINARY INFECTION

The marvelous filtering system present inside your kidneys has not been duplicated by man as yet. Not only do your kidneys filter well over a quart of blood each and every minute of your life, they extract the waste materials from an average of four and a half ounces of the serum portion of the blood each minute and deliver it as urine to your bladder. If you've been reading this book for about an hour, your kidneys have effortlessly filtered the wastes from more than 17 gallons of blood!

How Flushing Action Helps Your Kidneys and Bladder

In doing this filtering, your kidneys use a good deal of water. If water is in short supply in your system—if you're dry from working hard and not drinking much water—the cells in your kidneys simply concentrate your urine. They make it stronger by dissolving more waste material in a smaller amount of water. This does not strain your kidney cells as you might suppose. They're built to do this job. The only thing is that if this water supply gets low enough and for a long enough time, the more concentrated urine that results invites infection by germs that are present in your urinary system normally. The reason for this is that the concentrated nature of the urine is a good "growth broth" for germs because germs thrive better and grow faster in concentrated urine than in diluted urine.

For this reason, *using flushing techniques will prevent urinary tract infections better than any other single activity.*

Follow This Easy Routine for Flushing Your Kidney

1. The hotter the weather, the drier the weather, and the more physically active you are in such weather, the more you need to drink fluids.

2. As a minimum baseline, your kidneys should normally produce about an ounce of urine an hour. If it's been four hours since you last went to the bathroom, your bladder should contain a minimum of four ounces to maintain health.

3. Even under circumstances where physical activity and hot weather are not present, you should drink a minimum of ten ordinary drinking glasses of fluid a day. Anything that is in liquid form (pop, coffee, milk, juices) can be counted.

4. For hot weather, increase normal fluid intake by four glasses a day. For both hot weather and physical activity, *double* your normal minimum fluid intake.

5. In hot weather, some of your fluid intake may include cola drinks, coffee or tea. All these have caffeine in them that stimulate your kidneys to make more urine—and give better flushing action.

How Flushing Works for You

Flushing does two things: It dilutes urine, making it much tougher for germs to multiply in urine; and it washes out— flushes—millions of germs from your urinary tract each time your urine is passed. There are other causes for urinary tract infection and I'll touch on these later in this chapter. Meanwhile, *it's possible to prevent 85-90 percent of bladder and kidney infections by making use of flushing principles.*

CAN YOU STRAIN YOUR KIDNEYS?

I mentioned previously that you cannot strain your kidneys by making them work harder. Not more than a third to a half of the cells in your kidneys need to function under normal conditions—thus, always leaving a healthy reserve for any emergent situations that might come up.

The fact that more than this number of cells may be activated for one reason or another places no strain as such on a kidney. The fact that you may be putting off your flushing routine does not make your kidney overexert. It just brings more cells into action. Of course if there isn't any water at all (highly unlikely) for your kidneys to use, they don't make urine. Not because they've been strained, but only because they need water to dissolve waste products.

How Your Physical Toning Brings on Better Elimination

Physical exertion (where you actually strain muscles, for example) does present more waste for the kidneys to filter out. Any time your metabolism is stopped for any reason, there is faster breakdown of energy and nutritional elements (like carbohydrate and protein, for example) and more waste to dispose of. This stimulates your metabolism. Such physical strain is all the more reason to pay attention to your flushing routine, so that there is plenty of water for the wastes to be dissolved in.

How to Protect Your Urine Reservoir

The more fluids you drink, of course, the fuller your bladder becomes. Your bladder is a simple, hollow, muscular organ designed to act as a reservoir for urine from your kidneys. You feel it when it's full. When you feel it's full, it should be emptied as soon as possible so that the germs ordinarily contained in the bladder don't have a chance to multiply and grow. Once you start your urine, the bladder automatically empties itself completely so that less than a teaspoon full of urine remains inside the bladder after urination. I'll talk later about conditions that hinder this emptying out of your bladder.

HOW TO HAVE HEALTHY KIDNEYS

The work of your kidneys is actually quite complicated. Besides the filtering out of waste products there is actually a stage inside the kidneys where virtually all the dissolved chemicals in your blood serum (except for protein) is actually filtered, the wastes removed, and the chemicals your body needs refiltered back into your blood stream.

Good Health Principles Makes Better Kidneys

In addition, the cells that line the filtering tubes inside your kidneys have the ability to dump more or less salt, more or less sugar, more or less of about any of the blood's elements into the urine. These cells are under the control of hormones from your endocrine glands—they "tell" the kidneys what to do and how to do it. Another reason for reaching health control as soon as possible—the bonuses are staggering. Better kidney control is one of them!

When you sleep, you usually notice the urine you pass the next morning is rather strong or, in other words, concentrated. You've been sleeping for seven to nine or more hours without drinking fluids—your kidneys simply concentrate your urine.

A Good Rule of Thumb

Drink at least a full glass of fluid at bedtime (*after* your nightly toning routine is a good time) after you've emptied your bladder (just *before* your nightly toning routine). This will insure that the bacteria (germs) in your urinary system do not have a chance to multiply during the night.

HOW TO ACHIEVE COMMON SENSE ACID-BASE BALANCE

Your kidneys control your body's acid-alkaline (base) balance. The balance is kept constant by means of the kidneys' retaining or excreting into the urine the necessary salts that maintain the balance.

HOW ALMA CONTROLLED TOO MUCH ALKALINE

Alma U. is typical of many women I've seen with recurrent

urinary distress that seems to hinge on the acidity or alkalinity of urine. Alma was in her 30's and seemed to have two or three urinary infections each year. Investigation of the urinary tract didn't reveal any thing out of line. It was noted, however, that her urine tended to be quite alkaline most of the time.

By adding vinegar (acetic acid) in doses of one teaspoonful three times a day dissolved in water or juice, *or* by taking two tablets of Vitamin C (ascorbic acid) three times a day, Alma was able to acidify her urine just enough so that the germs causing her trouble couldn't grow and multiply so rapidly in her urinary tract.

FOLLOW THIS ROUTINE TO MAINTAIN ACID-ALKALINE BALANCE

To test your urine for acidity or alkalinity, you need some litmus paper. A piece of litmus paper (normal color: light blue) is simply dipped into a specimen of urine. If the urine is acid, the litmus paper will turn pink to red; if alkaline, the paper will stay blue or become a darker blue. Litmus paper can usually be obtained at any drug store.

These rules may help you with urinary irritations when it is based on a too acid or too alkaline condition:

1. If your urine is unusually acid (pink to red on litmus paper) during the day, you can alkalize it by taking one teaspoon of baking soda twice a day in water.

2. If your urine is unusually alkaline (dark blue on litmus paper) you can correct this condition as Alma did.

3. Keep in mind that the first urine specimen in the morning is normally a little on the acid side; while during the day and especially after meals, it is slightly alkaline. Such shifts are normal and need no correction.

HOW TO AVOID KIDNEY DAMAGING INFECTIONS

Your kidneys are susceptible to infection elsewhere in your body. Particularly they are vulnerable to the germ responsible for strep throats. This means that the sooner you have strep throat treated, the sooner you take steps to protect your kidneys.

I've discussed the problem of tonsil infections in youngsters. The same applies to adults. If you keep having throat infections, ear infections, or other infections caused by a strep organism, it is best to do everything necessary to have the source of such infection eliminated—your tonsils removed, for instance, in the case of strep throats, or have any bad teeth pulled, etc.

HOW TO START YOUR KIDNEY PROTECTION PROGRAM TODAY

To protect against infection, and hence, possible kidney damage, the following principles should be followed:

1. Keep after health control! Review all previous chapters for this important regulation.
2. In the colder seasons, get adequate rest and avoid pushing yourself to the point of fatigue, especially in cold, snowy weather.
3. Take special care of youngsters when they have one of the common childhood diseases (measles, for example). Strep infections are notoriously common on the heels of measles, mumps and chicken pox.
4. During any infection or during any process that causes elevated temperature (fever) double your fluid intake, even if you can't eat.

CHANGING A SLUGGISH BLADDER TO A HEALTHY ONE

Your bladder goes along usually functioning well until something upsets the balance. Then "all heck" breaks loose. Being a muscular organ, your bladder gets its full measure of tone by filling up with urine, then being emptied at the proper times.

HOW WALT OVERCAME BLADDER DIFFICULTIES

The bladder's tolerance for punishment can best be emphasized by a man named Walt W., who I once saw in the emergency room of a hospital. It seems that Walt had let some prostate trouble go and it got to the stage where his urine simply wouldn't pass out of his bladder. This situation had been present for about 26 hours by the time Walt had gotten around to doing something about it.

I drained about six quarts of urine from Walt's bladder which I could see protruding up into his abdomen about two inches above his navel!

As long as your bladder doesn't have to work against something below its outlet, like an enlarged prostate gland, for example, it does admirably well. Over the long haul, however, anything it has to push against to get the urine out will cause parts of its wall to weaken—something like a weak spot in an inner tube—allowing it to develop pouches that trap urine within them and are predisposed to infection.

HOW CATHY OVERCAME BLADDER "LET-DOWN"

In Cathy B.'s case, on the other hand, though there was a similar situation to Walt's—her bladder was having to push against a resistance below its outlet—it was caused by something entirely different. Cathy was much younger than Walt (she was 40, he was 65) but she had borne five children. As a result, she had worn down, stretched and otherwise weakened the supports of her bladder so that instead of being held fairly upright in her pelvis (this is the normal position in both male and female) it had been allowed to sink way back in her pelvic cavity, kinking the bladder's outlet. Her bladder had to push hard to get the urine out. Cathy also noticed that when she sneezed or coughed, she would dribble a little urine, a very embarassing situation for her.

In both cases, the patients had failed to keep their bladders in good tone by proper exercising. In Walt's case, this lack of tone didn't bring on his prostate trouble, but after his trouble was remedied, he failed to help his bladder recover. In Cathy's case, her trouble was the direct result of not paying attention to the preventive aspects of bladder trouble. I'll talk more about the care and treatment of the prostate in a minute. First let's see what Cathy could have done to help prevent her trouble.

FOLLOW CATHY'S PROGRAM FOR HEALTHY BLADDER TONE

1. Way back when she had her first baby, Cathy should have got her weight under control. She was 15 pounds over ideal weight to begin with, but with each succeeding pregnancy, she put on from eight to ten pounds to her baseline weight. When she was through having her family, she was 45 pounds overweight!

2. She was allowed to gain too much weight during the time of her pregnancies. No woman should put on more than 20 pounds total weight during the entire course of her pregnancy. Many women should gain no more than 15 pounds. *I've even seen a few women who should have continued to lose weight during the entire course of their pregnancies!*

3. Cathy should have practiced general muscle toning, but in particular, should have done special bladder toning exercises. This would have tightened

and strengthened her bladder supports and would have helped prevent her from gaining flab in her pelvis and abdomen.

Here Is a Special Routine for Females to Help Strengthen Their Bladder

1. Get into the knee-chest position on the floor (both knees drawn up toward the chest as far as comfortable, rump up in the air, resting your weight on knees and bent forearms).
2. Now make the muscles surrounding your vagina and rectum contract vigorously. You can do this by "sucking in" your rectum and vaginal muscles. Done properly, you can feel your rectum and your vagina contract from the inside—feel them both pull inwardly. This should be repeated—contracting and relaxing—for five to ten minutes.

This exercise should be done in conjunction with sit-ups, scissor kicks and scissor clamps (see Chapter 16).

The exercise for male bladders is much the same except it's done sitting on the toilet and consists of forcefully contracting the rectum. When done properly, you can feel your rectum pull inwardly and the muscles of your lower buttocks pull as well. The inward movement should be held for a few seconds, then relaxed. This should be repeated for five or ten minutes.

HOW TO AVOID KIDNEY STONES

Of the afflictions that affect your urinary system, renal stones (kidney stones) are the most painful. *And most of them can be prevented simply by adhering to the fluid intake principles I've discussed in Chapter 4.*

Most kidney stones are quite small, though they feel to the person who has one as big as the Rock of Gibralter. They're formed in the collection compartment of the kidney and are usually carried down the tube leading from the kidney to the bladder with the urine current. When a stone reaches this tube—called the ureter—it starts to cause trouble because the sensitive lining inside this tube reacts violently to such solid foreign material.

The severe colicky pain results from strong contractions in the ureter trying to force the stone down and into the bladder where it usually causes no further trouble. Generally, if you can tough it out through this journey from kidney to bladder, there is no further trouble since the small stone can usually be passed from the bladder to the outside during urination without difficulty.

What Happens with a Hang-Up

When a stone gets "hung up" along its downward course through the ureter, however, it becomes a problem. The stone must be removed because it obstructs the flow of urine on the side involved. A urologist usually passes a special type catheter up the bladder through the ureter and catches the stone in a "basket" on the end of the small catheter and then withdraws it. Occasionally, this doesn't work and surgery must be resorted to.

YOU CAN PROFIT FROM THE STONE PREVENTION PROGRAM

You can go far in preventing stones by adhering to the following principles:

1. Always take in ample fluids. Always drink more fluids in hot weather. Always drink even more fluids—up to double or triple your usual basic intake if your work is heavy and physical.

2. Pay careful attention to weight control and physical activity. Of the so-called "stone formers" I have seen (people who seem to have one stone after another), 80 percent of them have been overweight by considerable margins, and have had sedentary jobs. They had become lazy in both their jobs (weight control and physical activity), through paying little or no attention to health control!

3. Replace salt if you lose it through perspiration or hard, manual work. Your kidney can't use salt in forming urine if you're losing it by sweating faster than you replace it. Such salt loss is thought to predispose one to kidney stone formation.

4. Ask for an analysis of the stone if you pass one. Knowing the chemical composition of the stone can guide your medical advisor and you in preventing another.

A "STONE FORMER" ACHIEVES GOOD HEALTH

Cleve C., a middle-aged man I know, became a "stone former." He'd passed four stones in a two and a half year period. I met Cleve after he passed the fourth stone, and I had a chemical analysis done of it. The stone proved to be composed of chemicals of a strongly alkaline nature—the salts in it were precipitated out, in other words, in a highly alkaline (basic) urine. Cleve was also 45 pounds over ideal weight; worked as a plant pathologist for a pharmaceutical company; got little exercise; and drank too much alcohol. In other words, Cleve was quite short on health control.

Cleve reduced the 45 pounds excess weight. He began physical toning routines. He increased his fluid intake and reduced the amount of alcohol he took in. (Alcohol, among other things, dehydrates your system of water—it ties up water in its metabolism and takes it out of circulation.)

By taking in a little of one of the common antacids before and after meals, the particular salts in his kidney stones were prevented from being absorbed in such high quantities into his system. Cleve hasn't had a kidney stone now in ten years. And he isn't likely to as long as he maintains his body at top running efficiency.

HOW TO TAKE CARE OF YOUR PROSTATE

The male has a globe shaped gland lying just outside the exit of his bladder called the prostate gland. This gland literally surrounds the first part of the tube that conveys urine from his bladder to the outside. As long as this gland functions properly, there is no problem, and you never know you have a prostate. But let it act up and there can be trouble galore!

Inflammation—a Trouble Maker

Inflammation is the most common affliction of the prostate gland. You might compare this to what happens during inflammation of the tonsils—when they are inflamed they get enlarged, irritated, sore, and sometimes infected as well. The prostate becomes inflammed from a variety of causes—irritation; too much or not enough sexual activity; infection (such as venereal disease); tumors and the like. When your doctor does a rectal examination, he can feel the underneath surface of your prostate gland to see whether it is enlarged or normal in size—the prostate gland normally produces a slight bulge through the front wall of the lower rectum.

How Massage Helps

When the prostate gland becomes inflamed, the part of the gland that can be felt through the rectal wall enlarges noticeably and the gland becomes quite tender. Your doctor usually recommends prostatic massage if this is the case. This is done by "milking out" the congested prostate. He simply takes his gloved finger and presses down on the gland beginning at the top of the gland and sliding his finger down toward the bottom. This maneuver empties the gland of its excess secretions.

These secretions are passed into the urethra—the tube leading from the bladder to the outside—where they flow out the penis. The massage also stimulates the circulation in the gland and helps diminish inflammation. If the secretions appear to be infected as well as increased in quantity, your doctor may prescribe rectal irrigations of warm water and perhaps an antibiotic to kill the germs.

HOW YOU CAN KEEP YOUR PROSTATE WORKING SMOOTHLY

I once talked to a young man in his mid 20's named Hal F., who disproved the often heard declaration that "It's impossible to get too much sex." He came to my office with his prostate gland engorged to at least twice its normal size. It was so enlarged it was shutting off the flow of urine from his bladder. He had to literally squeeze out his urine and it was acutely painful to do so. In addition, he was running a fever of 101 degrees and had pain in both hips—a common site of pain with prostate trouble.

In talking with Hal, I found that he was a person who needed to constantly prove his manhood—he needed to be the living counterpart of a virile male stud. As a consequence of this need, Hal was having intercourse with as many as five women a week—more than once with some of them. This proved to be his prostate's undoing. It became enlarged, swollen, painful and infected. Hal's case responded to massage, antibiotics and cutting down on his sexual contacts. Some enlargement of his prostate persisted so I taught Hal how to do his own prostatic massage.

THE SELF-HELP PROSTATIC MASSAGE ROUTINE

Hal got hold of some rubber finger "cots" at his drug store. These are thin rubber tubes that fit snugly over the finger. Three times a week, Hal put one of these finger cots on his right index finger, gently inserted his finger into his rectum about an inch and a half, and milked down his enlarged prostate gland. *Gentleness* during the procedure is essential. If you press down too hard, it is painful and just irritates the prostate further. Done gently once a day or every other day and until the gland comes down to size, however, it can save your prostate from future trouble. Some vaseline on the finger cot may help in passing through the rectum.

For heat, Hal found that filling an ordinary enema bag with warm water, inserting the nozzle of the enema hose about two inches into his rectum and letting the water run in slowly and back out again worked quite well. The object here isn't to "take an enema," but just to deliver the warm water to the part of the prostate gland that bulges through the front rectal wall. If the tip isn't inserted too far, the water will run in and then back out into the toilet again.

Here Is How You Can Recognize Telltale Signs of Prostate Trouble

1. Diminishing urinary stream size, with increasing force necessary to get your urinary stream started.
2. A feeling you never quite empty your bladder even though you've squeezed out all the urine you can.
3. Dribbling urine later after you've urinated. Especially with physical strain or coughing.
4. An increasing feeling of fullness in your rectum. Any of these symptoms or any of the symptoms Hal noticed should get you to your medical advisor so he can help you with the problem.

On the opposite end of the scale from Hal, I've known several people whose prostate trouble began because of no sex contacts at all—some clergymen who lead celibate (no female contacts) lives, and who do not release their sexual tension by masturbation constitute the main category here.

Since there is no practical way to avoid this kind of problem and since so many people have set ideas against any sort of sexual relief such as masturbation, I've found that such patients eventually need surgery to relieve their symptoms, which are like Hals, except that they aren't so acute and persist over weeks or months at a time.

So it would seem that a happy medium, a middle-of-the-road attitude in sex is the best line to follow with regard to your prostate.

HOW TO ENJOY GOOD HEALTH FOR YOUR CERVIX AND UTERUS

The reproductive glands of the female are the seat of a great amount of trouble. I'm impressed that in women who have failed to take proper care of their general health such troubles are almost certain to present themselves sooner or later.

CLAIRE'S CERVIX PROBLEMS AND HOW SHE SOLVED THEM

You may find Claire E.'s case familiar. Claire was 47, married, and the mother of four children. She had slowly put on weight over the past few years until she was about 35 pounds overweight. She was active—a large family tends to keep one that way—but had failed to do proper toning to keep her physique solid and lithe. Instead, Claire found her muscles flabby and her abdomen protruding.

Soon Claire noticed that her urine was harder and harder to control—she would lose some every time she'd strain or cough, and she felt as though she didn't quite empty her bladder completely when she went to the bathroom. In addition to this, Claire was aware of a progressive feeling of fullness in her pelvis, "as though everything were slipping down and out," as she put it. Her bowels became more difficult to move, though she wasn't really constipated.

An examination showed the suspected trouble. Claire's pelvic organs—her uterus and cervix—had indeed "slid down." They were, in fact, beginning to bulge into the back of her vaginal canal. This had in turn allowed her bladder—usually well supported in front of the normal uterus—to be bent (allowed to fall) backward. Claire was past the help of toning or of weight reduction to assist in her own cure. Her pelvic organs were going to have to be removed or Claire could never have control of her bladder again and she would soon have her pelvic organs protruding from the mouth of her vaginal canal.

After surgery, Claire was convinced that she did indeed need to do better with health control. She went on a diet and lost 43 pounds over six months. She began toning. She concentrated on her protruding abdomen and found sit-ups and scissor clamps ideally suited to tighten up her lax abdominal and pelvic muscles, and return the support to her pelvis which she had lost through childbirth.

Within a year, Claire had perfectly normal bladder control, a figure more like the one she had when she was 25 years old, and she enjoyed perfect health.

You Can Reverse the Stretching of Childbirth

Childbirth does stretch pelvic organs beyond their normal limits. To avoid Claire's trouble, they must be restored to normal, and this takes attention—more than ever—to the principles given earlier in this book: Good physical and mental tone and the reduction of weight back to, *or* below, what your weight was before pregnancy.

MENSTRUATION AND HOW YOU CAN RECOGNIZE TROUBLE WITH IT

The following list will assist you to determine when menstruation needs to be checked into:

1. Bleeding *between* your usual periods.
2. Bleeding *after* sexual intercourse.
3. Severe pain with periods—real deep seated pain, not just menstrual cramps.
4. Profuse bleeding (instead of normal five or six day bleeding that tapers off after second or third day of flow).

All of these signs need checking into by your medical advisor. Don't hesitate to have it done if they appear.

HOW TO HANDLE VAGINAL INFECTIONS

The female vaginal canal is peculiarly susceptible to two main infections: Monilia—otherwise known as yeast infection; and Trichomonas—otherwise known as "Trich."

How to Recognize Yeast Infection

Yeast infection is characterized by the onset of vaginal discharge where there was only a minimal amount before, and by intense itching inside and outside your vaginal tract. Yeast is prone to come on during pregnancy and after a long session during which you've been on antibiotics for any reason. It is quite curable by any one of several methods your medical advisor can use.

How to Recognize Trichomonas Infection

Trich infection is caused by a small, one-celled organism normally found, but usually not productive of symptoms in, the lower bowel. It is thought that when women clean themselves following a bowel movement that if the habit is to move the toilet paper from the rectum toward the vagina, these organisms might be introduced into the vagina. At any rate Trich produces a thick, greenish foamy discharge that can be recognized instantly. It is treated by an oral medicine that makes quick work of the organism in about ten days.

Sometimes, the male sexual partner of a woman with Trich may get an infection in his urethra—the tube leading from the bladder to the outside. If so, he also can be treated with the same medicine.

Neither infection is considered serious—merely an uncomfortable nuisance. Neither causes harm nor are they likely to become future problems except that they may come back again any number of times.

WHAT TO DO ABOUT VENEREAL DISEASE

Venereal disease is on the upswing in this country today. No one can do more than guess just how much of an upswing because physicians traditionally refuse to report the majority of their cases. It's estimated that for each case that is reported to the public health officials in a given locale, there are probably at least 12 to 15 others that go unreported.

Why VD Is Up

In this day and age of sexual freedom among adults as well as youngsters, it behooves us all to be much more aware of this problem. VD risk is made even greater by more and more reliance on "the pill" and on the IUD for prevention of pregnancy—a fact which tends to blind most people to the VD risk. The old fashioned condom or "rubber" that the male used to prevent pregnancy had its drawbacks, certainly, but unfortunately its less frequent use today is a major factor in the rise of VD.

Playing It Safe After Contact

There is virtually no way you can tell for sure if a sex partner has VD. Therefore, if you believe you may have picked it up from someone, it's the safest thing to report in for examination at any one of the many VD stations run by the public health department in both large and small cities. Lacking such a facility, any medical advisor can do the examination and the treatment if it proves necessary. And it will be kept in the strictest of confidence.

The Domino Effect of VD

Remember also that any good VD control program has, as part of its operation, the case finding aspect. That is, if Henry Smith reports in with gonorrhea—a condition he may have first noticed as an increasing yellow-white drip from the end of his penis—and he is treated, the public health officials are quite interested in knowing where Henry picked it up—who he got it from, in other words. Because if this one woman from whom Henry picked up his gonorrhea can also be treated and cured, it's quite possible she may be prevented from spreading her gonorrhea to as many as a dozen or fifteen other men—and these men prevented from spreading the disease to untold numbers of other women who then may spread it to who knows how many others!

This then, is the reason for the reporting. You never know how many others you may save from VD.

HOW TO RECOGNIZE VD IN THE MALE

The typical case of gonorrhea in the male is characterized by a creamy, yellow-white discharge (drip) from the penis that is usually irritating and may cause discomfort on urinating.

Syphilis appears first and foremost as a single sore on the shaft of the penis that is not tender; looks like a shallow ulcer; and may disappear within a ten day or two week period. *This is the stage in which syphilis needs to be treated.*

HOW TO RECOGNIZE VD IN THE FEMALE

Gonorrhea is very difficult to detect in women because there is no striking appearance of the creamy drip seen in men. It may only be evidenced by a slight increase in vaginal discharge. A smear made by your medical advisor needs to be done to demonstrate the germ under the microscope.

If there is no direct evidence that the germ is present, but the suspicion remains, treatment is sometimes recommended anyway as a precaution.

Syphilis is the same. The painless ulcer may be completely hidden from view inside the vaginal canal. The second stage of syphilis occurring some weeks later may be characterized by a skin rash over the trunk and body that resembles any other rashy skin condition. The disease can still be treated at this stage. And it needs to be!

So if there's any doubt in your mind at all, any slight suspicion in your mind that VD is present, have your medical advisor or the public health clinic look into it. It will save you untold amounts of grief! And VD is easily treated and permanently cured.

SUMMARY

1. Urinary infections and kidney stones can be prevented for the most part by following a few important rules of fluid intake. This, supplemented by what you're already doing through health control, will help keep both from happening to you. Remember that bleeding from the urinary passage always requires expert help.
2. The bladder is generally neglected until trouble starts in it. You can keep your bladder functioning well and efficiently by preventing pelvic organ problems from entering the picture (women) and by keeping your prostate in a healthful condition (men).
3. The female cervix and uterus are the seat of much unnecessary trouble. Good physical tone, weight kept at ideal for height and frame, and periodic checks are the safe way to prevent this kind of trouble.
4. VD is on the rise in this country. It can be prevented by the more widespread use of the old fashioned condom (rubber), but the modern approaches to pregnancy prevention often keep this device from being used. High levels of suspicion, prompt seeking of treatment and diagnosis, and detailed reports on sexual contacts to Public Health Departments are the only good measures for VD control under present day circumstances.

8

How to Promote a Vigorously Healthful Digestive Tract

Your gastrointestinal tract—from your gullet to your rectum—is probably one of the most consistently abused systems in your body. You should know how to take care of your stomach and how to prevent ulcers and what to do about them if they occur. Your small intestine is the prime digestive area in your body— where most of your nutrition is absorbed. This organ needs proper care. You'll discover aids for this care in this section.

Your digestive glands—the gall bladder and pancreas—are an important part of your digestive system. They will come under consideration in this chapter.

The large intestine serves an important water absorption function and is the area where the normal bacteria of your body do their important work. You should know how to care for, and treat disorders for this important organ.

Piles are both a nuisance and a common affliction. You'll find ways and means of dealing with them in this section.

HOW TO TRAVEL THE PATHWAY TO A HEALTHIER STOMACH

I've mentioned previously how sometimes your mind, in its attempt to sidetrack emotional stress, will channel such energy through the large nerves that run from your brain to your intestinal tract. The first hint of trouble in this situation is either stomach cramps or acid stomach.

Cramps

This feels like someone put a rope around your stomach, knotted it, then began to pull on it. Cramps usually come along in waves—that is, they hurt painfully for a short time, then let up, though there may still be some pain between the waves.

Acid Stomach

Acid stomach, or acid indigestion, as some prefer to call it, is a definite heartburn type distress high in the center of your abdomen. A burning sensation is present which may at times be painful as well. It is usually constant, rather than in waves, and may also be characterized by belching up of "bitter gall" followed by a burning sensation in your gullet.

HOW YOU CAN FOLLOW RICK'S EXAMPLE
IN OVERCOMING STOMACH UPSET

A patient named Rick G. illustrates someone with both these distressing stomach disorders. Rich was 27, nervous, and bottled up things inside a lot. He was 29 pounds over ideal weight and tended to drink heavily, though certainly not an alcoholic by the usual standards. He smoked three packs of cigarettes a day. Here is the routine that stopped Rick's belly problems:

YOUR BEST PROGRAM FOR CRAMPS AND ACID STOMACH

1. Health control with weight reduction; 75 percent reduction in smoking and "explosion" physical activity when something or someone bothered him. This is the same technique used by Clark and Tim in Chapter 6.
2. Rick learned to sense his attacks coming on. When he felt one coming, he trained himself to lay down and concentrate on his stomach, repeating the phrase, "My stomach will relax" over and over again.
3. For the acid attacks, Rick took either three tablets of Milk of Magnesia or three teaspoons of the same preparation. He repeated this as necessary.

Within a year, Rick was hardly bothered by any stomach problem whatsoever, and was able to stem an attack when he felt one coming on. Today he is healthy and happy in the knowledge that he has acquired a powerful tool for stomach control to keep him in health.

How to Use Antacids as a Tool for Stomach Disorder

Antacids are quite useful in treating stomach disorders. I find most people do not use enough of the preparation or use it too infrequently when they do use it.

Milk of Magnesia, a common laxative, is also an excellent antacid. If you have to take only one or two doses in a 24 hour period, it is an excellent neutralizer of acid stomach conditions. If taken more frequently, it may also act as a laxative. If you're constipated as well, this of course, is the desirable thing to do. If not, then one of the non-laxative antacids is indicated. There are many such antacids to be found on the shelves of any drugstore. None of them has any advantage over the next, and all are equally effective if the directions on the container are followed. Whether you use tablets or liquid is only a matter of preference.

In a pinch, you can use baking soda for relief of acid stomach. The dose is one or two level teaspoons dissolved in water or skimmed milk. You should *not* continue the use of baking soda over any length of time since the antacid in baking soda is absorbed into your system and may upset your acid-base balance (see Chapter 7). None of the antacids from the drugstore shelf, including Milk of Magnesia, are absorbed—they act only inside the gut and can be used in much higher amounts over prolonged periods of time with safety.

How to Control Gas and Bloating

Excess gas is a most common disorder. The cause is invariably some food or group of foods that for you are difficult to digest. The cure lies in finding out which foods for you are the offenders and then eliminating them from your diet.

Some Foods That May Be Culprits

This list will help you if you have this trouble since it contains the common foods that are known to cause gas and bloating.

1. All fats. This includes the fat on all meats; whole milk; cream; cooking fats (drippings from bacon and other fried foods); and shortening. All oils as well—cooking as well as salad.

2. All fried food. It's the grease from frying that seems to be the offender here.

3. Beans; onions; cabbage; relishes; cauliflower or any preparation containing any of these foods. Virtually all spices and condiments (catsup, mustard).

4. Pastries, most rich desserts, and sweets.

HOW TO MODIFY STOMACH-IRRITATING EATING HABITS

Most people I know have atrocious eating habits. As I sit in restaurants or watch people at home eating a meal, I marvel at the ability of their stomachs to deal with such constant abuse. I'm talking about the person who bolts down his food, half chewed, and then rushes off to get wherever it is he is going. Sure, your stomach is tough, but there is a limit to what it can take.

Follow This "Better Eating" Program for More Efficient Health

These habits should replace your present ones and should regulate every meal you eat:

1. Chew all food thoroughly. Digestion begins in the mouth—give your nutrition a break.
2. Relax at mealtime if at no other time in your busy day. If you can, prop your feet up in a chair or on a table and concentrate a little on relaxing before you start eating.
3. Put all else out of your mind except for pleasantries—shove the job, the problems, and the rest out of the way if only for 20 or 30 minutes.
4. Don't be in such a rush! Slow down and take your time eating. When you've finished, continue to sit there and relax for ten or fifteen minutes—doze a little if you can.
5. Stop gorging yourself. You eat too much anyway. Stop short of feeling "full" and allow your stomach to begin shrinking a little. This helps with diet and weight control too!
6. Drink ample fluid with meals (with one exception that I'll talk about in a minute). Digestion is more efficient in liquid surroundings.

HOW TO TREAT YOUR STOMACH AFTER SURGERY

Valerie K. is a woman in her late 30's and had to have stomach surgery for ulcers. They had to remove about 60 percent of her stomach and clip the two large nerves leading to the stomach that cause it to contract and pour out acid. Following the surgery, Val noticed she had difficulty—it seemed that after every meal she would start to feel nauseated, weak and dizzy, and would often faint or vomit. All this in spite of her excellent recovery from surgery, complete lack of former pain from ulcers, and an otherwise good picture of health.

What caused this? Had surgery failed her? Val was having what is commonly known as the "dumping syndrome." This is caused by the sudden dumping of a normal meal into the small intestine, the meal finding no more stomach to reside in. Val was worried. She stopped all these distressing symptoms, however, by following two simple rules:

Your Best Bet for Health Following Stomach Surgery

1. After stomach surgery, *do not take fluids of any kind with meals.* (This is the single exception to the rule I talked about previously.) Drink your fluids *between* meals.
2. Eat six smaller meals a day instead of the one or two gigantic meals common to most eating habits.

These two rules will usually control the dumping syndrome quite satisfactorily.

HOW TO PREVENT AND TREAT ULCERS

We've already talked about how your gut may be used as a sounding board for emotions that are not dispelled—and I've talked about ways to handle such emotion. Nevertheless, an ulcer will form at times.

About 90 percent of stomach ulcers aren't in the stomach at all, but are located in the first part of the small intestine just beyond the stomach. This part of the small intestine is called the duodenum. Hence, 90 percent of what are called stomach ulcers are actually duodenal ulcers.

FOLLOW DON'S SUCCESSFUL ULCER TREATMENT PROGRAM

Don Y. came to me with his ulcer well entrenched. He was 42, married and in a high pressure type job. Don was also a worrier. Nothing was ever done quite to Don's satisfaction, and he stewed and fretted about such things all day and all night. More than this, Don used alcohol to quiet his nerves. He wasn't an alcoholic, just a little heavy on the booze.

Don's trouble first began with persistent heartburn about two hours following meals, and seemed relieved for a short time by eating. His extra eating to quiet his stomach put on about 40 extra pounds for Don over the course of about two years.

Still Don did nothing about the increasing, sometimes incapacitating pain which now was beyond the heartburn stage—it really racked him up at times. Soon it progressed to nausea and vomiting, especially after drinking alcohol to relieve his nerves.

Don then made the near fatal mistake of increasing his alcohol intake for the distress. He hemorrhaged from his stomach suddenly one night and was brought to the hospital in shock. Here is the schedule that stopped Don's troubles cold:

Seven Steps to Counteract Ulcers

1. Stomach constantly bathed in mixture of antacids and milk. Half and half type milk (half milk—half cream) seems more soothing in the case of an ulcer even though it's certainly not conducive to weight loss. At first this was done through a tube in Don's stomach; then in about two days he could take it by mouth without difficulty. Don took his half and half every hour.

2. Graduated diet—strict, then moderate, then liberal ulcer diets over the next six weeks. (Consult Chapter 16 for examples of such diets.)

3. Large doses of antacids—either two to four *tablespoonsful* of liquid antacid, or six to eight tablets. A third of the dose taken before meals; two thirds of the dose after eating.

4. The same dose of antacids three times a day *between* meals, and at bedtime.

5. The same dose of antacids at any other time heartburn or pain occurred. Especially if Don awoke at night with pain.

6. No alcohol. Cigarettes cut by 75 percent.

7. Health control started.

Don was in the hospital only two days and wouldn't have been there at all except for the bleeding episode. Fortunately, most people have their ulcers under control before such complications set in.

Following a six week period in which Don's ulcer healed completely, he pretty much ate what he wished except for the food he cut out to lose weight. He took antacids on an *on call* basis—that is, when he felt distress in his abdomen or had a case of heartburn. There have been no recurrences of Don's ulcer and no complications. There won't be if Don continues to master health control and takes care of his stomach.

HOW TO SHAPE UP YOUR SMALL INTESTINE

The final digestive phase takes place in the small intestine, and all the nutrition from the food you eat is absorbed into your system. You can begin today to make things much easier on your small intestine by setting up a roadblock on all that nervous energy which your body may be channeling into this organ, retarding its effectiveness and causing irritation—maybe even ulcers.

It is into your small intestine also that the digestive juices from both your gallbladder and your pancreas are poured after each meal. This function is automatic and will take place without your controlling it.

Five Points Program for Better Digestion

Your intestine will treat you better when you follow this advice.

1. Cut down sharply on your fat intake. A lot of fat causes bile to enter your small intestine in large amounts. Fat also puts on weight eventually and this, in turn, puts you at high risk for gallstones. Also, some vitamins are poorly absorbed in the presence of fat.

2. Chew meat, cheeses, poultry and fish well before swallowing. Digestion of proteins begins in your stomach and is completed in your small intestine. The easier you make things for your stomach—the easier your stomach makes it for your small intestine.

3. If you find foods (and almost everybody does) that disagree with your small intestine—cause gas, bloating, and crampy pain two or three hours after a meal—*eliminate these foods entirely from your diet.* Your digestive glands will last a lot longer and do a more efficient job if you don't push them.

4. The idea of smaller, more frequent meals will make your digestive organs and small intestine more efficient for you.

5. If you've had a lot of alcohol before a meal—like a dinner party, for example—don't eat nearly as much as you usually do and lean heavily on the protein foods such as lean meat.

HOW TO PREVENT GALLSTONES

A special word about gallstones. It happens there is a special type person who is very susceptible to gallstones. Nora W., a Midwestern farm housewife, was such a special type. Nora was married, of very fair complexion, and 42 years old. Over the years, Nora had let her health control go astray and when I saw her she was 63 pounds over ideal weight. She had always been in perfect health and when I mentioned her weight, she seemed somewhat irritated that I considered her too fat.

At any rate, Nora refused to do anything about her weight

problem. "After all, Doctor," she said, "why should I? Am I not the picture of health?"

How Nora's Weight Affected Her Gallstones

Within a year and a half of her last visit to my office, I was summoned to the hospital emergency room where I found Nora writhing in agony from severe belly pain on the upper right side, a fever of 101 degrees, nausea, and continuous vomiting for several hours. She'd also noted her stools were very light in color—almost milk-white—for the past 24 hours.

To make a long story short, Nora should have done something about her weight problem because people who are fair, fat and 40 are, indeed very susceptible to having gallstones.

Nora required immediate surgery because a large gallstone was lodged in the tube leading from her gallbladder to her small intestine. Her bile couldn't get through so it backed up and would soon cause damage to her liver if not removed.

The episode did make a believer out of Nora, however. She did bring her weight down to normal and has remained healthy since. She has not passed any more gallstones. Another of the many, many reasons, as I've repeated so often in this book, *for keeping that weight as close to ideal as possible!*

HOW TO CARE FOR YOUR VITAL LARGE INTESTINE

The last eight or ten feet of your intestinal tract comprises the so-called large intestine. It has one prime function—*to reabsorb fluids* from the already digested and mostly absorbed food delivered earlier to the small intestine. The contents of the large bowel begins as almost a pure liquid mixed with the undigestible left-overs from your food. By the time it reaches the rectum, most of this fluid has been reabsorbed back into your system and a soft pliable stool remains for excretion.

The way to treat your large intestine is exactly the same as you do your kidneys. *Always insure plenty of fluid intake each day.* This is because your large intestine will absorb fluid *at the expense of your stool*—you may be passing dry, hard, constipated stools simply because you don't take in enough fluids to keep them soft and pliable.

How to Deal with Constipation

It seems constipation is world-wide and always present to some degree in every household and in almost every person at some time in his life.

FOLLOW THIS EASY PROGRAM FOR SMOOTH BOWEL PASSAGE

The following is a list of common things that provoke constipation.

1. Not enough fluids.
2. Lack of abdominal muscle tone.
3. Not enough fluids.
4. Lack of bulk in diet.
5. Not enough fluids.
6. Nervous gut syndrome.
7. Not enough fluids.
8. Laxative habit.

The Role of Bulk

To add bulk to your diet, you simply need to eat more lean meat, more vegetables and fruit, and more whole grain cereals. This bulk gives your bowels something to work on to form normal stools.

The Role of Nervous Gut

The cure of the nervous gut syndrome lies with your channeling excess nervous energy. You've now had demonstrated to you thus far in this book several lines of attack: explosive exercise to rechannel emotional excesses; concentration on relaxation of the muscle wall of your intestine; concentration on the blocking of the nerves to your intestines; and training your bowel to move at specific times and intervals.

I once had a patient named Dudley I. who had been taking laxatives routinely for over sixteen years. He was convinced he could not move his bowels without them, and further, would surely succumb if he didn't take one or more laxatives every day.

How Dudley Overthrew the Laxative Habit

Dudley was the classic picture of "laxative habit," but even so it can be and was cured. Again, health control was started. Dudley hadn't exercised much during most of his life. It was difficult to talk him into it, but finally he tried. He felt so much better he continued and expanded his physical activities.

Dudley also concentrated each evening just before dropping off to sleep on this phrase: "My bowels will be active tomorrow morning." He repeated this phrase over and over. Within a couple of weeks, Dudley was having regular bowel movements each and every morning. He also increased his fluid intake about double over the usual for him. Within three months, Dudley was off laxatives altogether and hasn't had to use them since. He adds bulk to his diet by eating a bowl full of whole bran each morning. It works like a charm!

HOW TO BEAT CRAMPS AND DIARRHEA

Cramps and diarrhea are also common afflictions of the intestine. It's sometimes confusing to try and tell serious diarrhea from the relatively harmless types. The following table will help you sort out the different types of cramps and diarrhea:

HARMLESS TYPE	SERIOUS TYPE
Hits suddenly after previous good health. Lasts 24-48 hours at most.	Develops slowly but painfully. Past experience usually shows its presence before. May be chronic.
Seldom produces more than 4-6 stools a day. Watery and loose. Normal color to stool.	May produce 10-12 stools a day. May contain large amounts of blood and/or "pussy" looking material.
Usually not accompanied by chills or fever of note. May feel weak but not prostrated.	May have severe chills, fever of note (above 101 degrees) and may be incapacitated generally by illness.
Stools, though loose and runny, look normal.	Stools may be frothy, bulky or foamy and extremely foul-smelling.

Your Program for Stopping Diarrhea

For the harmless type diarrhea, you can usually treat them best simply by adding more fluids to your diet (to replace that lost in the watery diarrhea) and by using one of the solidifying agents of which there are several. *Plain* Kaopectate is one such and can be had at most drug stores without prescription. Most people, I find, do not use enough of these bowel tighteners. Take an ounce to two ounces (two to four tablespoonsful) at a time. Repeat half this dose after each subsequent loose stool that may follow. These preparations act only inside the gut—they are not absorbed and cannot possibly harm your system.

If you suspect one of the more serious types of diarrhea, you will need the help of your medical advisor. Don't hesitate to consult him if you need to.

Cramps usually accompany diarrhea. Sometimes cramps are there without loose stools; sometimes loose stools are there without cramps. Cramps usually disappear when the diarrhea stops.

How to Deal with Cramps

Cramps occurring suddenly and getting progressively worse with distention of your abdomen (protruding—swelling up), and with no gas or stool passing from the rectum *are a danger sign and must have the services of your medical advisor!*

If your bowels become too bulky, a low residue diet may help. If not bulky enough, a high residue diet may help.

MAKING USE OF WHAT IS AVAILABLE NATURALLY

There are also some natural laxatives that may help a constipation problem. These natural foodstuffs help soften your bowels and furnish your system with nutrition at the same time. They have the advantage that they don't cause you to become dependent on them—they can't become habits. A few of these follow:

1. Borcherdt's Maltsupex
2. Prune Juice
3. Sauerkraut Juice
4. Whole Bran
5. Fresh Fruits
6. Brewer's Yeast Tablets

I mention Borcherdt's Maltsupex here because it is one of the most versatile natural laxatives and is safe even for babies. Besides, it's nutritional as well, being a good source of B vitamins. Most drugstores carry it or can get it for you, and it doesn't require a prescription. Simply follow directions on the container. Don't hesitate to use more if necessary.

How to Watch for Appendicitis

Amazing though it may sound, appendicitis, if left untreated, racks up a terrific toll even in this day and age of miracle drugs. If you have any reason to suspect appendicitis in someone else or yourself, you should consult your medical advisor without delay. The following table will help you decide when to suspect appendicitis:

SUSPICIOUS	NOT LIKELY
Pain begins first, before other symptoms.	Other symptoms begin first, then pain.
Pain usually begins in mid abdomen, then migrates to right lower side. May be crampy at first, then changes to increasing *steady* pain.	Pain difficult to localize. Usually crampy type.
Low grade temperature elevation is common—99 to 100 degrees.	High temperature is uncommon until the late stages of appendicitis.
Nausea and vomiting usually occur *after* the pain starts.	Usually the reverse.

Appendicitis can begin after a bout of the grippe in which cramps and diarrhea may occur at first. But the picture changes if appendicitis enters the picture—the pain gets steady instead of crampy; it increases in intensity; and it usually localizes itself to your right side, generally low but can be in the middle or even the upper side.

Appendicitis is a surgical condition—its only cure lies in having it removed. If you wait until it ruptures, the picture is bleak. One word of caution: appendicitis can be very tricky in older people. For some reason the pain associated with appendicitis in older people is far less that it is with younger people. Therefore, in any older person (beyond 65 years of age) be very suspicious of vague abdominal distress with fever, nausea, vomiting, and signs of prostration.

HOW TO DEAL WITH PILES AND FISSURES

Piles (hemorrhoids) are varicose veins of the rectum. Most people have piles—some have trouble with them, others don't.

When veins lose their fibrous outer covering, they become varicose veins—they protrude through the surface. This is what makes piles. The veins normally present underneath the mucuous membrane of the rectum lose their fibrous coat and they protrude.

Sometimes they get irritated and bleed; other times they simply stick out through the rectum and become a mess to keep clean, itchy, and uncomfortable. They're seldom painful.

This Program Will Help You Deal with Hemorrhoids:

1. Take a hot bath in about four inches of piping hot water (the so-called Sitz Bath) or allow your shower stream to run directly on the hemorrhoids, as hot as you can reasonably stand it, for about five or ten minutes. This will help shrink them up.

2. After you move your bowels: *Always* hold pressure on any protruding hemorrhoids after you've cleansed your rectum. Use three or four layers of soft toilet tissue with three or four of your fingers holding very firm pressure against the protruding piles from below. This is best done with your weight shifted to one of your hips on the toilet seat—the hip opposite the hand you're using for the pressure. Move your fingers such that the protruding hemorrhoids are thrust back up inside your rectum, then hold pressure for a few minutes longer.

3. While holding this pressure on hemorrhoids after moving your bowels, do the same exercise I described in Chapter 7 regarding the bladder—"suck" the rectum up hard and hold it; relax; repeat this several times.

4. Following the pressure take a clean double sheet of toilet paper and squeeze on about a two inch strip of Vitamin A and D ointment from the tube. This preparation is available in drugstores without a prescription. You can also use Zinc Oxide ointment (as readily available as Vitamin A & D ointment), or you can mix the two for the best results.

5. Keep your bowels as soft and pliable as you can—avoid constipation as this condition only aggravates hemorrhoids. Here is a special exercise that a lady named Ona W. found quite helpful in shrinking her hemorrhoids, when used in conjuction with the routine I just described:

HOW ONA CLEARED HER HEMORRHOIDS

Ona stretched out on the floor in the same position as though she were about to do push-ups—weight supported on her extended arms and feet, legs and knees straight, with feet preferably braced against something solid like a chest of drawers, for example. Then she began a series of rotations (twisting) at her hips—first to the left, then to the right, keeping her legs straight and her arms and hands solidly planted on the floor. She rotated her hips as far in both directions as she could, straining for a little more rotation each time. This was repeated several times, then repeated again, this time letting her arms bend a little, bringing her body closer to the floor. Again, she repeated this rotation, this time with her hips elevated—her rump thrust higher than her head. This was done for five to ten minutes twice daily.

Ona had excellent results with this routine. In about a year and a half, she was rid of her hemorrhoids completely.

One note of caution: Any hemorrhoid that develops *sudden severe pain* in it means that it has become thrombosed—has formed a blood clot inside it. To relieve this quite painful condition, your medical advisor will have to evacuate the clot. It is a simple office procedure and the relief you feel will be worth any trouble you may have to go to.

How to Fight Fissures

A fissure is simply a painful crack in the skin around the rectum. It's usually partly outside and partly inside the rectum. Every time you move your bowels with a fissure, it's painful.

The same ointments can be used to advantage with fissures as I listed before with hemorrhoids: Vitamin A & D ointment and/or Zinc Oxide ointment. These preparations should be applied to the rectum after each bowel movement and before retiring at night. You may find that the help of a finger cot—a small rubber tube that fits over your finger—is helpful in applying the ointment to the part of the fissure inside the rectum. It is important to keep the bulkiness of your stool as low as possible during the healing of a fissure. (Refer to the low residue diet again in Chapter 16.) It's also important to keep from becoming constipated during the healing. Sitz baths often help. If after two weeks, your fissure isn't healed, some help from your medical advisor will be needed.

There are many suppositories made for hemorrhoids and fissures. However, the above mentioned ointments are all you need. You may use any of the many suppositories available to add to your therapy, but use them along with the ointment—you'll have better luck.

SUMMARY

1. You owe it to your stomach and small intestine to practice the principles of good care and feeding to prevent ulcers, nervous stomach cramps, and heart burn.
2. Your digestive function can be made to operate smoothly and effi-

ciently, and your gallbladder and pancreas do their jobs easier if you follow all the principles of health control.

3. You can start today helping your large intestine perform its job by paying attention to fluid intake, diet, and the way you live your everyday life.

4. Piles and fissures can be dealt with uniformly good results by using techniques of heat application, ointment application, and bowel function principles.

9

How to Regain and Retain
Healthier Skin and Teeth

Your skin, exposed as it is to the total environment, bears quite a lot of the brunt of wear and tear. You will want to discover how to help your skin stand up to these onslaughts so as to keep this most important covering of your body healthy. We'll also have a look at leather skin and wrinkles and what to do about them in this section.

The ever present problems of pimples—their treatment and prevention—will come under discussion here as well as bags under the eyes and double chins.

In this section we will examine the much overdone problem of fungus infections on the skin, and other skin infections and sores that may develop on your skin.

Also, the problem of moles and how to tell the good ones from those that are potentially harmful is covered.

Your hair and teeth, being products of your skin, are reasonable targets for total health. You'll discover how to prevent balding, cavities, and what will and won't keep your hair and teeth from falling out.

HOW YOU CAN COPE WITH WRINKLES AND LEATHER SKIN

What to Do About Wrinkles

I suppose I have never attached the deep seated significance to face wrinkles that I should—I've made a lot of patients mad because I failed to get all worried and unstrung because of the presence of wrinkles on their faces. I think a few wrinkles on your face are both natural and desirable—a few give a look of maturity and wisdom to your countenance. A look, I might add, that will enrich and enhance your own personality if you'll only look at them in this light.

I'll agree that too many wrinkles on your face does age you a bit, and too many wrinkles can and should be avoided.

There are four main sources of too many wrinkles and leather skin: the sun, the wind, excess fatty tissue, and lack of facial muscle tone. The effects from all four can be prevented or greatly minimized.

Obviously, facial muscle tone and the presence of too much fatty tissue in your face have already begun to be corrected—or have they? You *are* paying attention to your face in regard to your toning routines? You *are* bringing down that weight? If not, I want you to read Chapter 2 again with special attention to the toning of your face. This should be a regular part of your toning routines. Losing weight down to ideal levels will automatically take off facial flab. It won't just hang there in folds *if you do proper toning of the facial muscles at the same time.*

I've recently heard some plastic surgeons decry facial exercises as causing more wrinkles—as not being good for your face. I disagree. Unless you are a movie star whose ego can't stand the slightest blemish on his body, I feel that in the long run you'll fare better doing them (facial toners) than not. I urge you to at least try.

How to Control Leather Skin

Leather skin is the product of sun worship among people who don't really have to be in the sun, and among people whose jobs keep them in the sun and wind most of the time.

Eventually, and each person has his own particular tolerance, the sun simply dries up all the skin's ability to produce oil. It dries up. Leather skin results. So the way to deal with this distressing outcome is to prevent it from happening in the first place. The single rule is simple: If you *have* to be in the sun, take extra measures to apply a good sun screen (tanning or burn preventive) at least two or three times a day. This also applies to not-so-sunny but windy weather as well. If you have nothing else, plain vaseline liberally applied to all exposed skin will work well against wind and cold weather.

Protection from the sun requires a sun screen ingredient in either an oil or cream base to filter out the ultraviolet rays that do the damage. The most effective sun screen for these rays is a chemical called para amino benzoic acid. You might check the list of ingredients of the liquid anti-sun preparations on the drug counter to get the best protection.

A GOOD PROGRAM THAT WILL HELP YOU AVOID WRINKLES AND LEATHER SKIN

1. If you're going to expose any portion of your skin to the sun—even for a tan, use an effective *sun screen* preparation two or three times daily. When you wash your face next, use a mild soap—with nothing added to make you smell better—and then rub some face cream or hand lotion into your exposed skin.

2. When you rub in creams or lotions, take some time to massage the tissues while you are doing it—under eyes, chin, eyebrows, ears and nose. Don't forget your neck, forehead, and temples. And make certain you protect all these areas with your sun screen and vaseline.

3. You women go easy on make-up. Use as little of it as you can reasonably get by with.

BERNICE CONQUERS FACIAL ECZEMA FROM MAKE-UP

Bernice Q. wondered, for example, why she had chronic eczema on her face. She'd been to three doctors and had three different medicines prescribed for her inflamed facial skin. None of them worked. She was beginning to show chronic permanent changes in the skin around her forehead, eyelids, and upper cheeks when I saw her.

In questioning Bernice, I found she was in the habit of using eyebrow liner, eyelash liner, "pancake" make-up of unknown quantities, and a host of other things to make her more attractive to the opposite sex. In reality, all she was accomplishing with this movie make-up bit was to sensitize her skin to a variety of chemicals in all these various compounds. Her skin was crying for relief.

When I finally convinced Bernice that she should stop using all this junk and stick to the basics of good skin care, her chronic eczema cleared up completely.

Soaps and Deodorants Are Hard on Your Skin

We've all, to some extent, been guided into habits the manufacturers of various products would like us to use. One of the most common skin agers I know of are the soaps that have deodorizers and all sorts of chemicals added to do this or that. It is best to keep these off your face, particularly if you're beginning to show signs of wrinkles or leather skin. The chemicals are sensitizing and really dry out what remaining oils your skin may have left. The result is a hastening of skin aging. Use instead, any *plain soap*—one that has nothing in it but mild soap. And use this sparingly except for conditions I'll come to in a minute.

HOW YOU CAN HANDLE PIMPLES, ACNE, AND THEIR COMPLICATIONS

When I talked before about leather skin and wrinkles, I've been talking, of course, about mature adults who have passed adolescence. In the time of life between mid and late teens, however, the problem is exactly the opposite—the surging power plant that takes over an adolescent body overdoes almost everything, including the production of excess oil in the skin. This is the basis for pimples and acne. It's also the basis for preventing trouble—your aim to dry up this excess oil.

YOU CAN HELP YOUR ACNE AS ED DID

Ed T., a small town high school student had just turned 16. He began to blossom out with pimples all over his forehead, chin, shoulders and back. He was getting a good start on acne.

He was concerned, as he should be, but had started using a variety of products his friends told him would cure his acne. Unfortunately, Ed's acne got worse over the weeks, and he was forming pus under many of his pimples which were beginning to run together on his face to form *rosettes*—clusters of pimples behaving as one big sore.

Using Ed's Program for Results in Acne Cases

1. *Diet.* If you want to reduce what already is too much oil in the skin of your face and upper trunk, you've obviously got to reduce to the absolute minimum all the known dietary sources of oil and grease. This includes all fried foods, all fats, all salad and cooking oils. It includes all foods containing *chocolate,* which also means all *cola drinks* since these drinks are all derived from cocoa beans. It includes nuts, candy and pastries, peanut butter, cream,

and butter. Ed found he didn't have to abstain from all these foods, but had to cut them by 90 percent to remain pimple free.

2. *Face washing.* Ed washed his face three times a day—lightly, so as not to irritate his face skin—but thoroughly. Soap dissolves oil and grease in the skin. Ed used plain Ivory soap.

3. *Drying lotion.* At night before bedtime, Ed found that by diluting either soap or shampoo (see below) with water, he could find the dilution that dried his facial skin yet didn't irritate and inflame his skin. He used this water-soap or water-shampoo mixture each night by patting it gently onto his face following washing, and then allowing it to dry right on his skin.

4. *Dandruff problem.* Acne and increased dandruff usually go hand in hand and the flakes from falling dandruff with their oils are sometimes enough to cause acne of the forehead, neck and shoulders. Ed found that a preparation called Fostex was an excellent shampoo to control dandruff. He did the first lather with plain soap, and used Fostex for the second lather. Twice a week was enough. When his dandruff was controlled in a few weeks, he cut down to once a week for washing his hair.

5. *Pimple control.* For pimples with pus or a yellow head, Ed pierced each one with a sewing needle soaked in alcohol to sterilize it. He didn't squeeze or press hard on each pimple—just opened it before washing his face and let them alone thereafter. For blackheads deep in his skin, Ed found that a soak with his washcloth and warm water opened his pores, and that blackheads eventually came out with washing or with the use of his drying lotion. Squeezing them, he found, invariably inflamed and worsened things. Simple drainage was all that was required.

Within six weeks, Ed cleared up 85 percent of his acne problem. Time and good sense with skin care and scalp care got rid of the remainder. Today, Ed's skin is clear, has no scars, and is healthy.

Short Hair and Electric Shaving

I recommend that hair be cut fairly short when acne and dandruff are present, and that you use electric shavers if you can possibly afford them. They are much easier on the skin and don't give it a bunch of knicks or cuts as straight edge razor blades do. For those who use a safety razor, use an unscented, unsmelly shaving cream to protect your skin as much as possible. Try and avoid cutting your skin through frequent blade changes and using careful technique—unhurried and without trying to solve several other problems during shaving.

HOW YOU CAN ELIMINATE BAGS UNDER YOUR EYES, AND DOUBLE CHINS

Bags beneath your eyes mean that your health control needs boosting. The skin beneath your eyes is rather thin anyway, and if the muscle beneath this skin—a circular muscle that surrounds the entire eye—is lax, fluid normally present in the tissues collects in abundance and puffs the skin out.

The eye exercise I discussed earlier in talking about facial tone is the beginning of unpacking such eye bags. This is done by closing your eyes forcibly and with pressure, and alternately contracting and relaxing this circular muscle. A finger placed below your eye will tell you if you're doing this correctly—you can feel the circular muscle bunch up. The exercise should be done for five minutes twice a day along with the other face toners.

Massage of the eye bags with any hand lotion or facial cream is then indicated following your toning routine. You should spend a couple of minutes briskly rubbing the lotion or cream into sagging or puffy skin each morning and night.

If you awaken in the morning with rather pronounced puffiness (common after a bad night with late hours and too much drinking) hold an ice cube firmly on the puffy area for about five minutes before the toners and cream massage.

Your Sagging Double Chin Techniques

In the case of extra chins, fat has collected in excess underneath your chin. This area tends to be loose anyway, and if your body weight is out of control, your chin is a favorite site to collect more than enough flab for one, two or even more extra chins.

The toner specific for extra chins is as follows: Drop your chin onto your chest. Now tighten up as much as possible on the chin muscles—use your entire array of neck muscles to do this if it's easier. Alternate contracting and relaxing these muscles ten times or more. Now, keeping your front neck and chin muscles tight, elevate your chin until it points toward the ceiling. Now thrust out your lower jaw, first to the left, then to the front, then to the right sides, all the while holding your front neck muscles tight. Repeat this ten or more times.

For a change of pace, get hold of a fairly solid rubber ball about six inches or so in diameter. Place it on a high table, sit beside the table, catch the ball under your chin and roll the ball around in a wide arc over the table top. Do this for five minutes two or three times a day.

How to Use Artificial Lights Properly

What about the heat and ultraviolet lights for skin conditioning and tanning? I've seen two patients who both had life-long grief from misusing ultraviolet and infrared lights to restore their skin. Wilma L., who overused ultraviolet light in the mistaken hope that she was going to restore youth to her facial skin, first presented herself to me with second degree burns on her face from overexposure. When the burns healed in about six weeks, she resumed the treatments—against my advice. Today, Wilma, at age 39, has a face that looks like 55 from leather skin—and she's stuck with it.

Buck D. thought to improve his pock—marked face (from previous acne not well controlled) at about 28 years of age. When I saw him about a year later, he had deep facial skin burns of a chronic nature from overexposure to infrared light. When he was forty, Buck had a face that looked like a story book gnome. It was as wrinkled as a dried up old prune. And beyond redemption.

I don't recommend either ultraviolet or infrared light to treat skin conditions of any kind. I have often recommended a plain 60 watt light bulb in a goose-neck lamp to help dry up any oozing, moist skin condition. Even this must be watched so that burns won't result, but I've never seen permanent damage or serious trouble from using it.

How About Hormones, Packs, and Facials?

About every two or three years, a new hormone turns up on the market in a cream base and which is to be rubbed into the skin (especially the face), and it's supposed to perform miracles. I've yet to see any such miracle. There are hormones that will temporarily smooth out face wrinkles when used as directed. The effect is only temporary, however, and their prolonged use will only *accentuate* the wrinkles and make them more prominent. Then there are all the fancy packs. I think I've heard of faces—particularly women's faces—being packed in virtually every-thing known to man. Including, I might add, cow dung. For all the expense of such packs (they go all the way up to 100 dollars for a raspberry pack) and for all their weird variety, I advise you to stick to the basics of skin health. The simpler methods are vastly less expensive and will do your face more good than all the facials in the world.

HOW TO TREAT FUNGUS-LIKE INFECTIONS

The skin is subject on occasion to fungus infections to be sure, but for every true fungus infection on your skin, you will have about ten other conditions—none of which are fungus infections.

What to Do About Swimmer's Ear and Athlete's Foot

Seen in the summertime or in warm climates where swimming is always in season, the condition called swimmer's ear is often attributed to a fungus. It isn't a fungus at all but merely an inflammation in the skin of the ear canal caused by dampness and not drying thoroughly after swimming. It can also occur from constant wetness that isn't dried properly from any source. A cotton wick soaked in one of several formulas listed in Chapter 16 will usually suffice to clear it up. You should not swim or even wash your ear canals until it's clear again.

The same thing can be said of athlete's foot—true fungus infection of the feet and hands is uncommon. Inflammation between the toes and fingers is commonly caused by inflammation of the skin which is the result of oversweating, dampness not dried well, and so forth. A true fungus infection generally starts at the root or at the sides of finger and toe nails; is chronic and characterized by redness, soreness, itching and scaling of the skin along with discoloration of the nail. A formula for keeping the skin of your feet healthy may be found in Chapter 16.

How to Deal with Canker Sores

Canker sores (also called cold sores, fever blisters) may occur on lips, chin, tongue and inside your mouth. They look like a white patch surrounded by a cherry red halo. They are painful and a nuisance. I've listed the best formula for this condition in Chapter 16. Canker sores always clear themselves in time.

YOUR GUIDE FOR HANDLING SKIN WOUNDS AND SORES

Your skin is subjected to hundreds of cuts and abrasions throughout life. Considering their sheer numbers, it's surprising that more of them don't get infected and cause trouble like the hand cut Donna got one day. She had what looked like a simple, shallow cut with a knife. She got it as she was slicing frozen hamburger in the kitchen one day. She thought no more about it when it stopped bleeding.

When I saw her five days later, Donna was running a fever of 103 degrees, was having chills, and had red streaks running from the small wound up her arm to her shoulder. The lymph glands at her elbow and under her arm were swollen and tender. Donna had what is commonly called blood poisoning from an infection getting into the small wound in her hand.

This kind of trouble can be prevented by treating all cuts, lacerations, abrasions and the like as though they might get to the stage Donna's did. With your wounds properly treated, Donna's troubles won't happen to you.

FIVE POINTS TO REMEMBER IN DEALING WITH WOUNDS

1. Scrub all wounds, big and small, with plain soap and warm water as soon as you can.

2. Keep a bottle of hydrogen peroxide in your bathroom. Irrigate all such wounds with this excellent germicide after cleaning with soap and water. Just take off the lid and pour the peroxide right into the wound from the bottle. If the peroxide doesn't foam and bubble in the wound it means it's lost its potency and should be replaced with a new bottle. Peroxide is quite inexpensive and can be had without a prescription at any drugstore. It's the best antiseptic I know of.

3. Cover the wound with a simple dressing—clean gauze, band aids or whatever. If you notice redness developing around the wound, pus in the wound, or red streaks flaring out from the upper end of the wound, you need help with its care from your medical advisor.

4. If you can't get to your medical advisor right away, and you see signs of blood poisoning as Donna did, start the hot towel treatment immediately. This is done by securing at least two hand towels, soaking both in a large pan

of water simmering on the stove. Wring out one of the towels slightly and completely wrap the wound with the hot moist towel and the area for several inches above the wound as well. As this towel cools down, replace it with the one soaking in the water and throw the cool towel in the hot water for continued use. Keep this up for about 30 minutes three or four times a day. This activitiy may keep the infection contained and from turning into blood poisoning.

5. With all scrape wounds where dirt is ground into the wound, even though it appears to be quite shallow: *Always take a clean brush and scrub out the dirt from the bottom of such wounds.* If you fail to take this precaution, you can expect the wound to gather pus almost every time. Scrubbing hurts. It makes the wound bleed. But do it anyway. You'll save yourself much trouble later on!

HOW TO COMBAT BARBER'S ITCH

Duane came to me with a severely inflamed face. It started the day before, following his usual morning shave with a safety razor. His facial skin was vivid red and hurt like the devil. It was beginning to form pus on the surface. The process was limited to the whiskered area of his face. Diagnosis: Acute Barber's Itch.

Duane found almost instant relief from this common condition—generally seen in men who shave with blades—by using a compound called Quinolor ointment. This product can usually be found already made up on your druggist's shelf with the name Quinolor on the package.

YOUR MOLES AND HOW TO TELL A BAD ONE

The vast majority (99.99 percent) of moles are completely harmless and needn't worry you. One special type, the so-called *melanoma* has certain characteristics that should alert you to possible trouble. The mole may have been colorless or may have been the usual brown, but suddenly it takes on a slate-blue color, almost black, and if you look closely, there may be a halo of slate-blue or black color around the main mole. These need the attention of your medical advisor. All other moles are best left alone unless they are located in a place where your clothes irritate them all the time. These can be removed easily if they need to be.

Any mole that has been flat—as most are—but suddenly begins to take on a cauliflower look should also have help. I recall seeing one such mole in the navel of a man I'll call Frank. Frank had this mole as long as he could remember—probably from birth. It had never bothered him at all. It was right in the pit of his belly-button and looked a little like a piece of worn, brown leather.

One day, one of Frank's small children stuck her finger in Frank's navel and the mole bled profusely. Frank had it removed surgically and it proved to be a type of mole that often turns into a tumor. He was glad he was rid of it.

HOW TO DEAL WITH WARTS

Warts are another harmless nuisance. They're colorless, raised bumps anywhere on the skin, especially the hands for some reason, that occur after being scratched, bumped or bruised. They're caused by viruses in the skin and why the viruses cause warts, no one knows. Most warts will disappear by themselves if left alone. They can be removed easily if they're bothersome. A good wart remover is listed in Chapter 16.

I know people who have had their warts talked off by people especially adept at this technique. What a wart talker does is a carefully guarded secret and I haven't the foggiest idea how they do it. I do know that warts are peculiar in that they have a single, little artery going right up the middle of them and if this tiny artery is cut off by any means, the wart shrivels up and goes away. If you concentrate hard enough, you could cause this little artery to constrict and pinch off. Your wart would then go away. You'll have talked your own wart away.

YOUR BEST METHODS FOR ATTRACTIVE HAIR AND TEETH

Caring for Your Hair

Scalp hair arises from the skin on top of your head. Good principles of care for this area of the skin will be the secret to health so far as your hair is concerned.

People are concerned about balding. They don't like it when their hair starts to thin out or fall out. It ages them. There are a couple of very rare diseases that actually cause baldness. You won't run into more than one or two of them in a lifetime. I haven't seen such disease in a patient that I thought might be the cause for baldness, though I've seen plenty of baldness that had nothing whatsoever to do with some dread disease.

Take Clay M. for example. Clay was only 35 when he noticed his hair coming out by the gobs full from several patches on his head. He thought surely he must be dying of some unknown disease when actually he was the picture of health.

In talking to Clay, a rather common pattern of events came out which may help you avoid Clay's problem. Clay was used to showering almost every day. He always washed his hair when he showered and had for years. He used the same soap he used for his body to lather up his scalp the first time, then a popular dandruff shampoo for the second rinse. All this, of course, helped Clay have a dandruff-free head of hair, until it began to fall out. I also found out that Clay liked to wear the newer fancy bolero type hats with the feather sticking out the hat band and the narrow, zippy looking brim. It seemed to make Clay look more like a "man-about-town."

USING CLAY'S PROGRAM FOR YOUR FALLING HAIR

1. I asked Clay to stop wearing hats altogether. Sometimes the constant wearing of hats or caps can slowly constrict the scalp's blood supply (by the hat or cap's snug fit) just enough to begin to kill off the hair follicles—the tiny shafts in the skin of the scalp from which hair grows. When this happens the hair on the top and sides of the scalp may all fall, leaving a thin margin of hair on the lower head and around the ears.

2. I asked Clay to stop showering so much and to wash his hair no more than once a week. Further, I had Clay use plain soap (Ivory) for the first rinse and ordinary green soap for shampoo. Your skin anywhere is better off not being washed as often as every day. This tends to dry it out. Same with your scalp. In addition, many shampoos and bath soaps contain harsh chemicals that bleed your scalp oil glands, and hence, your hair, of its natural oils. Stick to the simple soaps and shampoos. They're easier on your hair and skin.

3. I instructed Clay to rub in the oil that shampooing removed. That is, to replace the lost oil by any good non-alcohol containing hair dressing—the kind that comes in tubes. Alcohol is drying and may cause hair to disintegrate.

4. Finally, I noticed some scaly red, patchy lesions in Clay's scalp skin, especially around the hair fall-out areas. He had a mild case of psoriatic-like affliction in these areas of skin. I had him rub Pragmatar ointment into these areas two or three times a week. This ointment is especially good since it is non staining and it washes right out whenever you want to do so. This

ointment can also be picked up in a package with the name "Pragmatar" on the container. If you can't find it, the formula is given in Chapter 16. I find that women have similar trouble when they over do hair sprays, hair sets, fingerwaves (permanents), and when using other various chemicals they insist on putting on their scalps and hair.

HOW HILDA STOPPED BALDING

A woman named Hilda T. for example, began her patchy baldness for no apparent reason she could think of. In talking to Hilda, I found out she was in the habit of rolling her long hair in curlers so tight it hurt, each and every night. She also was used to pulling her hair into either a tight bun or pony tail—again so tight it actually caused pain. Yet Hilda was willing to put up with this torture for the sake of being stylish.

When Hilda stopped using tight curlers, tight buns, and tight pony tails, her hair stopped falling out. It was that simple.

HOW TO HANG ONTO YOUR TEETH

Teeth are generally sadly neglected. Unfortunately, you only get two natural sets of them in your life, so the permanent set must be given attention or they're lost and gone forever.

When your adult set of teeth have all appeared—usually in your late teens or early twenties—they are especially subject to cavities and decay until you're about 35 or 40 years old. Then they usually behave themselves and cavities seem far fewer at this time. Your gums are what need your particular attention.

Proper Care of Your Teeth

It goes without saying that teeth should be scrubbed well, preferably twice a day, certainly once a day. This should be done with a fairly rigid toothbrush—one that will stimulate your gums as you brush. A soft, frazzled toothbrush just won't do the job. The scrubbing should be done first with a mixture of salt and soda—about half and half—and then with any toothpaste you like. The attention should always begin and end with your gums, not your teeth themselves. The gums should be vigorously scrubbed, from the top down for upper gums; from the bottom upward for lower gums. Both sides of your gums need scrubbing—the outside of them as well as the inner side, from the very back to the front, both upper and lower.

The best thing you can do for your teeth and your gums is to use dental floss regularly. Every night is not too much and at any other time you eat a meal with roast or baked meat or food containing coarse fiber—corn, cereal and the like, you should use dental floss. A piece of floss about nine or ten inches long should be torn from the container and wrapped securely around one of your fingers of both hands. This anchors it so you can push the floss between the spaces between every tooth in your mouth and give it a gentle sawing motion back and forth and from side to side to remove the food particles that get stuck there, and that you can't possibly get out with your toothbrush.

Good Dental Care Is a Must

Your dentist should be seen at least twice a year up to age 40, then at least once a year. This way cavities can be discovered and filled before they rot out your teeth, and the deposit of various salts that precipitate out in your mouth during meals can be scraped and chipped off before they produce gum irritation. After forty years, the dental floss routine and the scrubbing become all the more important even though your teeth seem more resistant to cavities at this time. Careful attention to these apparently simple details can save your mouth a lifetime of grief, and you may well have as many of your original teeth at age 70 as you did at 17.

Once in a while infection flares up in your mouth at the roots of teeth. An abscess may form. This means you need to review your teeth health principles again, and it also means you're going to need help with the condition. Infection (abscess) usually starts with sudden pain and swelling at the root of the tooth involved. It causes the face above the infection to swell and get puffy—sometimes the entire side of your face on the side of the infection swells up. Your dentist needs to be consulted immediately at which time he will probably put you on antibiotics for a few days. If your dentist can't be reached, then your medical advisor should start the antibiotics. Later, the involved tooth will probably have to be pulled.

Your dentist will then tell you again just what I've been saying about the care of your teeth. Pay attention! The teeth you save may come in handy some day.

SUMMARY

1. Wrinkles, leather skin, pimples, and acne can be prevented and success-fully treated. A little attention to weather exposure, together with common and inexpensive preparations will save your face from aging.
2. Control of eye bags and extra chins are functions of your already started physical toning. You may rid yourself of them by facial toners and keep them away by toning every day from now on.
3. "Fungus" infections usually turn out to be just skin irritations. Skin sores need principles of first aid diligently applied, to prevent infection, fungus or otherwise.
4. Moles are generally harmless and can be controlled. The harmful ones are easily spotted.
5. Your hair and teeth are items that respond and last you well and long if you take a little time to apply health control to them. You can save the hair and the teeth you started out with by applying such control today.

10

How to Put Strength and Zip into Ailing Muscle and Bone

Stiff, aching muscles and arthritis continue to plague our bodies in spite of medical advances. Both these aggravating conditions can be handled effectively. You'll discover how in this section.

Sprains and strains of joints and our old friend, back trouble, are also a source of much disability and discomfort. We'll talk about how to control both of these conditions in this chapter.

There are several tricks of the trade in handling the various forms of arthritis and foot ailments. You'll discover some of these tricks so that you may bring health control to bear on these areas.

HOW TO RELIEVE STIFF, ACHING MUSCLES

How to Control Muscle Spasms

When you overdo almost any muscular exertion, you may notice afterwards that a specific muscle may be stiff, and if you try to use it, it hurts. Sometimes, the stiffness gets so great that you couldn't make the muscle move if you wanted it to. What has happened is that the muscle has developed a spasm—the muscle cells remain contracted, pinched up—even though you tell it to relax.

The same thing happens if you overexercise certain muscle groups to the exclusion of others. For example, a weight lifter does too much bicep muscle exercise. He flexes his arm while holding a lot of weight, and neglects to use the bicep antagonist muscles, the triceps (the large muscle in the back of your upper arm). Soon the weight lifter's arm begins to hang with the lower arm permanently curled up. He has let his bicep muscle become muscle bound—get so stiff it cannot be relaxed.

149

This is why in Chapter 2, I mentioned the doctor's routine and said he had a good mix of toners—he used each of his muscle's natural antagonists as much as the main muscle itself. His muscles never got stiff.

YOUR STIFF MUSCLE ROUTINE

1. Use the stiff muscle, but don't exert it strenuously—take it easy, but don't baby it either.

2. Use heat. Use heat at least four times a day for at least 30 minutes. The stiffness will disappear almost in direct proportion to the amount of heat you use. Just be careful you don't burn your skin.

Whether you use moist heat or dry heat isn't too important. You can stand in a shower for instance, and let the hot water beat against a stiff, sore group of back muscles. You can soak sore hip muscles in a bathtub of water, keeping the water hot by replacing it often. You can use a heating pad or a hot water bottle on a stiff arm, or leg, or shoulder. When using heating pads and water bottles, it's best to pad the skin with a layer of flannel or a towel. You can moisten the protective cloth for better heat holding power.

3. Massage. Enlist the aid of another person or do it yourself. Lubricate hands well with mineral oil or any hand lotion, then begin to knead the stiff muscle, working from the middle of the muscle to the outside and from top to bottom with thumb or finger tip strokes (rubbing). Massage is best done before the heat and should not be so vigorous as to cause the muscle to hurt more—*gentleness* is the way. Firm but gentle.

4. As an alternate to heat use one of the medicated heat rubs. These chemicals cause the sensation of heat when rubbed into skin overlying the sore, stiff muscle by causing irritation. This increases the blood circulation which is what regular heat does. The same end point results. Above all, don't be discouraged. Keep up the steps above until results are achieved. The bigger the muscle, the longer it takes.

5. Use oil of wintergreen (also called methyl salicylate). Rub this into the skin overlying the stiff muscle after the massage, and before the application of heat.

How to Overcome Strains and Sprains

Strain means overstretching. I've just talked about sore, stiff muscles—this is a strained muscle. Sprains are more severe and require more attention than simple strains or pulls. The following signs will help you decide if sprain is present:

1. Rapid swelling—not slow as with more simple pulls or strains.

2. A feeling of warmth around the sprained area.
3. Much distress with moving the sprained part—not just mild discomfort as with pulls or strains.

A sprained area usually involves a joint such as an ankle or wrist or knee. A sprain usually involves torn ligaments without damage to bones (fractures or dislocations). Sprained joints should first of all be strapped to help immobilize them. If after strapping you still have considerable distress when the joint is used or when weight is placed on the joint (the ankle or knee, for instance), you should seek help from your medical advisor.

YOUR FIVE POINT SPRAIN MANAGEMENT PROGRAM

1. For swelling: Use ice packs for the first 48 hours. Ice helps resolve swelling which decreases pain quickly. Ice cubes can be put in a bread wrapper or other plastic wrap and placed directly on swollen areas. This should be kept up for 20 to 30 minutes four to six times a day.
2. After 48 hours: Heat applications will be helpful with pain and stiffness. It is easiest to use hot water for joints since they can usually be submerged right into the hot water. Other forms of heat are just as good but not as easy to use for most joints.
3. When strapping a sprained joint area, first apply compound tincture of Benzoin solution to the skin wherever adhesive tape is to come into contact with the skin. (This is the same solution that you use for inhaling for bronchitis and hoarseness). Allow to dry after painting on with paint brush or daubing on with cotton or gauze. Your skin will be greatly helped and will not be irritated by the strapping adhesive tape.
4. After you have strapped a joint, make it a point to elevate the extremity when sitting down—put your leg up on a chair or lounge if you have a strapped ankle, for example. If you're up—move around, but don't stand around in one spot.
5. Keep the joint strapped for ten days to two weeks. Change strapping if it's needed. If the strapping is uncomfortable, it *needs* to be changed.

If you have an active family, or you have growing youngsters at home, or if you live in the country, it's always wise to keep a pair of crutches around for use. You never have them, it seems, when they're needed. The best thing you can do for a severe injury to a leg, for example, is to get off the leg completely—use crutches to help you walk on your good leg, picking up the injured leg off the ground or floor entirely.

HOW TO MASTER STRAPPING TECHNIQUES

How to Strap an Ankle.

Start six or eight inches above the injured ankle on your lower leg and apply circular strips (one inch tape is easy to use) from above downward, toward the injured ankle. Make these strips firm but not too tight. Alternate circular strips from one *side* of your lower leg, extending around the injured area to the opposite side. (These will pass around the bottom of your heel from one side of your leg to the other.) Now apply some more strips of tape from the back of your heel forward along the sides of your foot (these strips will pass around both sides of your ankle, including the injured side). Then another vertical strip, just in front of, or just behind the first. Then another circular strip, then vertical, then horizontal, in that order. When you're finished, you will have the tape strips interlocking, passing over and under other strips in a basket weave fashion. This weaving strap method will hold fast if you're on your feet, and it will stabilize your injured ankle. It will also keep you from bending your ankle when walking.

How to Strap a Knee

Start with long tape strips—24 to 36 inch strips. Start in back of your lower thigh about eight or ten inches above your knee joint, and bring the long strips downward and forward in a spiral, making at least one complete turn of the strip around your leg. Try to avoid passing the tape over your knee cap—plan knee straps so that you'll end up with a small square of exposed skin over your knee cap. Then place a shorter vertical strip along the inside, then another along the outside of your knee joint. Then do another spiraling strip starting just below or just above the last. Then some more side strips, then some circular strips around the leg, above and below the knee joint. Then spiral, vertical, and circular until the knee is stabilized snugly.

You're aiming here for stability and to keep your knee from bending when you walk. If it bends, the strapping does no good. When you strap any joint on an arm or leg, the entire extremity should be brought up even with the waist or higher, so that you won't have swelling below the strapping when you're finished. It's always best to try and get the injury swelling to come down with ice *before* you strap.

How to Strap an Injured Chest

When you bruise a rib or crack it, strapping can be an aid in the pain such an injury causes. You'll notice that when you crack a rib, every time you take a breath, and on many movements you make with the arm or shoulder on the same side as the injured rib, it really hurts. What's the answer? To stabilize the side of the chest where the injury has occurred.

For this, you need a second person. Sit yourself down in a chair, leaning forward slightly. Have your helper plan to tape an area six to eight inches above and below the injured rib. The trick here is to use strips of tape one or two inches wide that extend from two or three inches beyond the center of the spine to two or three inches beyond the center of the chest *on the side of the injury*. When your helper applies the strips (after, don't forget, painting thoroughly with tincture of Benzoin) let all the air out of your chest and have him apply the strips *after* the air is let out. This way, when you're through you won't be moving the injured side of your chest much during breathing. And this will control most of your pain.

If the injured rib is on the person's right side, apply the first strip of tape about two or three inches to the left of his spine and bring it around over the injured area, then around to the front to about two or three inches to the left of his breast bone. After applying eight or ten strips above and below, as well as over the injured area, you've helped him a lot with his distress.

How to Strap a Back

There are a host of back strains, sprains, pulls and other injuries that can be helped with proper strapping. The object here is to create a girdle of adhesive strips well above and well below the site of the injury (just like with ribs, ankles and knees), such that it is difficult for the injured person to bend or stoop over, and so that the muscles involved in the injury are well supported in any position he assumes.

Start by applying several vertical (up and down) strips over and on either side of the injured area. Then apply horizontal strips of tape (side to side) above and below the injured area extending around so that the ends of the tape are just in front of the rib cage on both sides.

You may also intersperse strips that are diagonal (from right upper side to left lower side, for example) between these up and down, and side to side strips for the same "weaver" effect that you learned in strapping an ankle. When you have finished, the patient should automatically keep his back perfectly straight when sitting, standing, and lying down, if you've strapped it properly. This will help him feel much more comfortable while his back injury heals.

HOW TO MAINTAIN A HEALTHY BACK

The most common site of injury to the anatomy is your back. The more physical the job you do, the more apt you are to have a bad back every now and then; the more apt you are to pull ligaments and muscles in your back—usually your low back, though your neck and the area between your shoulder blades are also common locations of injury.

How to Combat Housewives' Back

I've given the name *housewives' back* to a very common ailment I see frequently among women, but men aren't exempt from having it as well. This injury typically begins with a housewife bending over to do something, feeling or hearing a snap in her lower back, and then being unable to straighten up again without severe lower back pain, or doing so with much distress. Typically, I find the housewife was bent over the bathtub washing out the ring or scouring the tub. Sometimes, she's bent over a low cupboard in the kitchen or over the clothes dryer removing the dried clothes.

However it occurs, it's very frightening and very painful if it happens to you. Your first thought is usually, "My God, I've broken my back" or "I'm paralyzed." Fortunately, neither of these disasters has occurred at all. What has happened is that in bending over, you've put a group of muscles and ligaments (ligaments are what hold bones together, as between the vertebral bodies in your lower back) and/or their tendons (tendons are the gristle that attaches muscles to bones) on the stretch. These muscles, ligaments, and tendons are the ones that bend and straighten up your back.

In the process of bending, you've overstretched them. They go into spasm, the same kind of strain and sprain type spasm I've already discussed. When the muscles that ordinarily straighten out your spine contract against their antagonists that have gone into spasm, sharp, severe, deep pain results. And though the discomfort is great, the damage is generally quite minimal.

What do you do with this condition? The best maneuver at first is to lie down on the floor or, if you can make it, in a well supported bed, and apply heat. You'll find that this gradually relaxes things enough so that you can slowly but surely straighten out your legs and get into a reasonably straight position again. Once this stage is reached, you can get someone to strap your back or you can get into a well-fitting corset or other similar foundation for back support. You can take three aspirin right away and two every two or three hours for pain relief.

YOUR PROGRAM FOR A HEALTHY BACK

1. Never, never bend over or stoop to get at something on floor level. You can train yourself to *squat down* to whatever it is you need to get at, grasp the object you need, *then use your legs again to lift you up. All the while keeping your lower back perfectly straight.*

2. Use a bed board in your bed between mattress and springs. A sheet of half or three quarter inch plywood is good for this. It should extend from about shoulder level to mid thigh level. Ordinary bed slats laid side to side also work well for this.

3. Use back exercises to strengthen your back when the painful injury is gone and you can do so without your back hurting. A good one to start with is the cradle rock. This is done by lying on the floor on your stomach, bending both legs at the knees, reaching back to grasp both ankles with your hands and starting a rocking motion using your abdomen as a rocker. Strive to rock forward to your face, then pull backward with arms and hands and at the same time straighten out your legs so you can rock backward, clearing your chest and upper abdomen from the floor. A few of these will be all you can manage at first. Gradually, as your back gains strength, you'll be able to spend several minutes two or three times a day at it.

4. Another method is to stand with one arm supporting you against a dresser or other solid piece of furniture, reach back and grasp your right ankle with your right hand, and try to straighten your leg, arching your back at the same time. The same with the left hand grasping the left ankle. Also the *peek-a-boo* exercise I described in Chapter 2 where with your legs spread apart about two feet, you bend forward and downward until you can see an object behind you—a lamp, for instance—then straighten up and bend backward at the waist until you can see this same object again. This, repeated

several times for several minutes two or three times a day will add back strength.

After you've strapped your ailing back, use dry heat—a heating pad or padded hot water bottle will do. Before you strap your back, your shower running vigorously on the sore area, turned on as hot as you can comfortably take it, is very good.

What to do with Serious Back Injuries

Not all back injuries are harmless. Perhaps you've had a serious one yourself or know someone who has. Here is a list of signs that will help you decide if a given back injury is serious.

1. The pain from a serious back injury usually does *not* limit itself to a particular area of your back. It travels. Usually into your buttock, into your thigh, and even into your lower leg. When this sign is present, you need help from your medical advisor.

2. Strains, sprains, and pulls usually heal in ten days to two weeks, particularly if you're following the treatment rules I've just talked about. Serious back injury does not get better in spite of these principles—it may linger unaffected by anything you do. Such lingering back pain—not responding in reasonable time—needs help. Don't hesitate to seek it.

3. After a fall, even from a short height, in which you land on your tail bone or rump then notice severe pain in your lower back—higher up than the part that contacted the ground—may mean you've damaged your bony parts. This calls for help. Try to stay put, in a chair or in bed until help can be obtained if this sign is present.

4. After any back injury, and after a reasonable time for healing, if you notice that coughing, sneezing, or straining (grunting, for instance, in passing your bowels) sharply aggravates your back pain, this may mean trouble. Seek help.

5. Finally, if you have any trouble moving either leg, foot, or toes, or if you develop peculiar sensations in either leg—like areas of numbness, prickling feelings or burning—seek help.

HOW THESE PEOPLE OVERCAME COMMON INJURIES

1. Ted S. twisted his ankle while slopping hogs on his farm. He noticed almost immediate swelling progressing to the point where his injured ankle was twice as big as his uninjured ankle. He also noticed a bruising effect over the bony point at the outside of his ankle, as though he'd been struck by a direct blow. His ankle was quite painful and strapping it didn't help. X rays of this ankle revealed a bone chip on the outside ankle bone. He thought he'd just sprained it.

Warning: A bruising sign after wrenching injury is almost always indication of bone injury. It looks like a black and blue collection in the skin overlying the area of injury.

2. Marvin L. fell to the ground during a high school football game—he'd been tackled. He twisted his right knee and heard a popping noise at the time. The knee was weak and sore, but he continued to walk around on it following the game. The next day, his knee was quite swollen, mostly on the inner side of his knee. He couldn't straighten his knee without much pain. He had a knee joint full of fluid and had injured both ligaments and cartilage in his knee joint.

Warning: Fluid in a large joint like the knee, and inability to move through the usual range of movement without severe pain should warn of internal joint damage.

3. An elderly lady named Nancy B. walked into the emergency room of the hospital saying she'd fallen at home, with her left leg forced outwardly. She'd noticed some pain in the area of her left buttock at the time, but later when walking noticed some pain mostly in her left knee. Her left knee didn't seem injured at all and wasn't swollen.

X rays revealed Nancy had fractured her left hip! Yet she walked to the hospital.

Warning: After an upper leg or hip injury, pain from an injured hip may be actually felt in the knee. Also it is sometimes possible to walk on a fractured hip, though if suspected, not recommended!

4. Bob A. was working on heavy construction. He fell into an open pit and landed on both outstretched arms. He noted some medium pain in his left wrist, though no bruising or deformity you might see with a bone injury. The most striking thing was stiffness and inability to move any of his fingers too well. Bob decided not to have it checked. Over the next four or five days, pain increased and stiffness of fingers became worse. On examination something was obviously wrong, though without swelling of great note, it wasn't thought to be more than a sprain. X rays revealed dislocation of all the bones of the wrist save for one (there are eight wrist bones).

Warning: Increasing pain and *increasing* stiffness of fingers after a wrist injury usually spells trouble.

5. After a minor blow to his upper front chest, Jerry F. was not alarmed. In two or three days, Jerry became aware of a severe knife-like pain sharply localized over the area of the blow. There was nothing unusual about the appearance of the skin overlying the blow, and his ribs seem quite normal. Pressure over the area made Jerry come up off the table with pain. He was convinced he'd "punctured something inside." What he really had was a minor displacement of the joint where the cartilage part of one of his ribs joins the breast plate—the condition is quite harmless, but extremely painful.

6. Barbara R., a rancher's wife, noticed increasing pain and distress in her lower back but could not date the start of the distress to anything she'd been doing or to any injury. The pain was fairly localized to an area midway

between the back part of the large flat hip bone and the middle of her back bone and was on the right side only. The pain didn't travel but sometimes it was worse when sitting or lying down, than it was when standing or working. It got neither worse nor better over several weeks' time.

Investigation revealed arthritic changes in Barbara's sacroiliac joint on the right side. Proper therapy relieved it altogether.

Warning: Pain that doesn't seem to fluctuate with what you're doing, and that may be as bad or worse when resting or lying down as it is when up and active, is an indicator of something wrong deep inside.

HOW TO HANDLE ARTHRITIS

The subject of arthritis has occupied more books, articles, and discussions and yet it is one of the least understood of all illnesses besetting the human being. Unfortunately, arthritis has also become the target of more ill-advised cures and medicines than any other I know of.

The reasons for all this are easy to see when you look at the natural history of this affliction. By this I mean that it is the natural course of all forms of arthritis to come and go. And if you're taking some odd-ball cure such as alfalfa and rhubarb at the time your arthritis is ready to get better anyway, the alfalfa and rhubarb will be given credit for the *cure*.

Arthritis is hardly ever cured. It is handled, controlled, alleviated. Hopefully, someone will find a good cure for it, but until he does we'll all have to be content with its control.

Dealing with Rheumatoid Arthritis

This is the arthritis of younger people. No one knows what starts it, though all kinds of guesses are made and every year someone comes up with a fancy theory. It may begin with simple swelling and mild tenderness of any one or several of the middle finger joints. It's characterized by its migrating habits—you may have it in your left elbow one week, in your right knee the next, and in your back six months later. Pain and stiffness are usual and swelling during the acute stage is not uncommon. When the process stops—and it always does eventually no matter how you treat it—the swelling and pain go away and some stiffness may or may not remain.

YOUR GUIDE FOR RHEUMATOID ARTHRITIS CONTROL

1. If one or more joints are red, swollen and painful, the joint should be kept reasonably immobile—should be put at rest, in other words. This stage is usually short-lived, a couple of days to a couple of weeks at most.

2. During this hot stage, all the heat you can give the joint (locally) is helpful—dry heat, moist heat, both kinds—just sock it to the area several times a day for 20 to 30 minutes.

3. Initially, during the hot stages of rheumatoid arthritis you will help your cause by starting large daily doses of any aspirin compound *and maintaining large daily doses of aspirin for at least the next three weeks whether or not the pain and stiffness remain that long.*

By large doses, I mean take three or four aspirin initially and two aspirin every two or three hours while you're up during the day. Sometimes this dose of aspirin makes your ears ring. Cut down the dose a little if this is so. Soon the ringing will stop. Also, such doses may irritate your stomach—give you heartburn or indigestion. If this occurs, take the aspirin with meals and/or with antacids like milk of magnesia or any of the other antacids you'll find on your druggist's shelf.

4. When the joint or joints cool off, that is, lose their warm feeling and redness and the pain subsides noticeably, *then begin to put the involved joints to work.* If the disease is in a hand, start squeezing a child's firm rubber ball several times a day for a few minutes; if a knee, begin to walk, cycle and so forth regularly; if a back, start toning the muscles in the fashion I've already discussed. This is to break up stiffness which tends to remain and become a little worse with each episode if you don't take steps to head it off.

5. If you are overweight, and if your bad joints are back, hips, knees, ankles, or feet, *start taking steps today to reduce your weight to an ideal level!*

6. Check, or have yourself checked, for any possible source of chronic infection anywhere in your body. Such sources of chronic infection, even though they may not bother you between bouts of arthritis, may well be the main source of the arthritic flare-ups. Teeth, tonsils, the female pelvis, and the male prostate are common sites for chronic infection, as well as the urinary tract and sometimes the chest. Such sources of infection can, and should be eliminated with the help of your medical advisor.

7. *Do not plan on changing your life style just because you may have arthritis.* Unless the change involves *more and greater activity,* that is. Keep your health control going at all times—you'll be happier and much less uncomfortable in the long run if you do.

8. *Do plan to try and avoid the acutely stressful situations that may be a part of your life patterns.* In regard to this last item—stress—I'm not referring to the strains and pains of everyday living. I'm talking about the real dangers in your life—the divorce, the changes of location by moving around the

country a lot, the "knock-down, drag-out" squabbles with the spouse and/or the kids.

In other words, when you've got rheumatoid arthritis, you can go through some changes in the way you tackle this business of life and at least get yourself in a position so you aren't apt to have to be "drug through the jute mill" every month, year in and year out.

HOW CAROL CONTROLLED STRESS,
FOR CONTROL OF RHEUMATOID ARTHRITIS

A lady in her mid 50's I recall named Carol V. found this out. Carol was a widow trying to raise three boys by herself. She was the sole support of the family, was not wealthy, nor was she made comfortable by a lot of insurance when her husband died. Her family life became one of constant bickering and argument with her boys who rebelled at the usual age boys do, only more so without the firm, guiding hand of a father. Carol began to have trouble at work and was threatened with the loss of her good job. At this time, Carol began her first bout with rheumatoid arthritis: swelling of the middle finger joints on both sides, painful left shoulder, stiff lower back and neck.

It wasn't until two years later that Carol found out what I meant by eliminating stress factors. At this time she remarried, fortunately to an intelligent, understanding man who took over both the breadwinning and the boy raising chores. Carol's arthritis virtually disappeared within six months of this change in her life, and to date has not recurred.

How to Deal with Osteoarthritis

Osteoarthritis is a degenerative arthritis and is seen in older people and in joints that have been severely injured in one way or another. It is different in that it doesn't show the swings that rheumatoid arthritis does. But it does have its good and bad times, only in a less pronounced way. The treatment is exactly the same as for the rheumatoid type except that for a joint—the hip, for example—that may eventually become useless, surgeons have devised means of completely replacing the hip joint so that the person can enjoy using his legs again.

Osteoarthritis seldom produces redness or warmth about the joint, but otherwise it is quite similar in feel to rheumatoid arthritis. It may start, as in the rheumatoid type, in your fingers, but in osteoarthritis, the terminal (end) finger joints may be the first to show bumps and pain, rather than the middle finger joints.

How to Deal with Gouty Arthritis

Gout is an unusual but not rare kind of arthritis that primarily afflicts men. It often starts with acute redness, pain, and swelling of the large toe on one foot. It may also show small bumps scattered around the body, mostly on the ears. So painful is this type of arthritis that it must be handled by special drugs that only your medical advisor can supply. Again, gout, like other arthritis, comes and goes, but with the newer medicines, can be held in more or less permanent check.

For some time, gout has been blamed on diet. Personally, I've never seen any striking result from going on the so-called "purine-free" diet, though many people seem to think it helps. If medicine therapy is properly applied, I think it is generally a wasted effort to try and stick on a diet for gout.

THE PROPER CARE OF YOUR FEET

The following is a list of common foot afflictions and how you can deal with them:

1. *Corns:* Found on pressure points from shoes and from adjoining toes. Should be filed or ground down to skin level—not cut or shaved. A pumice stone or nail file, after soaking corn in warm water will help do this. Areas of pressure should be eliminated. Use better fitting shoes, padding with moleskin, or felt with adhesive on one side and cut to size. These materials can be obtained from your druggist or surgical supply house.

2. *Blisters:* Acute rubbed-up areas beneath pressure points. Filled with clear fluid. These should be punctured with a sewing needle soaked in alcohol to sterilize them. Make puncture wounds at *base* of blister at several points around the circumference of the blister. Allow to collapse and protect the thin skin covering from being rubbed off by padding with band aid or corn padding material. If infected (redness, pus, red streaks running from blister) use a warm soak technique described in Chapters 3 and 4.

3. *Ingrown Nails:* This is usually on the big toe. Carefully pry

up the nail edge along side grown in, after thorough soaking in warm water. Cut out a triangular wedge of nail with clippers or razor blade, with the base of the wedge along the outer nail edge. If infected: Hot moist soaks several times a day, peroxide to clean, padding along outer and/or inner edges of toe.

4. *Bunions:* These are hard, bony projections from the outer side of the big toe. To cure they must be chiseled off by a surgeon or chiropodist. For relief: Padding with moleskin, or felt with adhesive on one side, and much wider shoe than you usually wear.

5. *Plantar Wart:* "Ingrown" wart, usually on undersurface of foot, near ball of foot. This must be dealt with by medical advisor since they don't respond to usual wart removers (see Chapter 16). For temporary relief: Padding with moleskin. Cut a hole from center of a round pad and place hole over wart. This spreads pressure from walking to areas other than over the wart.

6. *Fractured toes:* Usually will heal without much to do. Wear stiff soled shoes. Tape the injured toe to the one next to it if necessary. Pain may force you to get off the foot for a couple of days. You can accomplish this by walking on your heel or with the aid of crutches.

Foot bone fractures other than toes require medical advisor's help.

7. *Athlete's foot:* Scaling, itching, redness between toes with discoloration at base of nail. Soak in potassium permanganate solution three times daily for two weeks. Rub solid alum moistened with water over involved areas after soaking. Keep toes and feet dry by frequent change of socks; liberal use of any talcum powder dusted on skin and in shoes. Dissolve three to six potassium permanganate tablets in warm water for soaks.

SUMMARY

1. You can deal effectively with stiff aching muscles, charley horses, and pulled tendons and ligaments through use of heat, strapping, and aspirin, together with good sense in protecting the injured part by not using it.
2. Your back can be made healthy through strapping, heat, and strengthening muscle toners. When a serious injury occurs it will require help from your medical advisor.
3. Arthritis occurs in three common forms. Each can be handled, but not permanently cured, as a rule. Heat, rest and aspirin form the mainstay in

treatment of each form in spite of all the new drugs and hormones and in spite of the current fads brought forth for treatment. Your medical advisor should decide on any stronger treatment.

4. Care of the feet requires the sensible use of moleskin, or felt padding with adhesive on one side; soakings; and good sense with shoes and the treatment of any infection.

11

How to Cope with Headaches, Sinus Conditions, Eye Trouble and Nasal Difficulties

You will discover how to deal with headaches in this chapter. They are common, they are painful, and they can incapacitate. You should know how to handle them when they plague you.

An often blamed area for headaches are sinus cavities. You'll find means to recognize when sinuses are the cause for trouble and when they're not. They are blamed far too often for trouble caused by something else, but when they do give trouble, you should know how to head it off.

Your eyes are one of the most important organs in your body. They are exposed to a host of troubles. Their care and handling is important to you.

Your nose filters all the air you breathe through it and without good nose function, you can neither smell nor taste—try plugging up your nose and next time you eat a meal to get an idea just how much your nose plays in your enjoyment of food and awareness of your surroundings. Your nose is subject to troubles and you'll see how to deal with them in this section.

HOW TO DEAL WITH HEADACHES

For some people, a headache is cause for alarm. Actually, the fact that it may hurt is cause for some satisfaction. Why? Because the worst things that can go on inside your head you don't feel at least until late in the game.

Nerves and Blood Vessels Can Be Troublemakers

You can view your head as being affected by deeply buried structures and by structures fairly close to the surface. The deep structures in your head that cause pain are blood vessels. Anything that stretches blood vessel walls in the head causes pain. This is the cause of migraine headaches, for example.

An example of a close to the surface headache would be one caused by inflammation of sinuses. The majority of your sinuses are fairly close to the surface of your face. The two sets of sinuses that are more deeply set behind your nose have their own kind of symptoms which I'll talk about a little later.

Another sub-surface cause of headaches is nerve bundles that run beneath the skin of your face, neck and scalp.

With these structures, nerves, sinuses and blood vessels, you have the cause for 99 percent of all headaches. But what of the dreaded brain tumor? You might wonder. What of this serious producer of headache? The fact is that headache is *one of the last symptoms* produced by a tumor. There are many tell-tale signs that occur long before headache in the case of a tumor.

HOW TO DETECT MIGRAINE HEADACHES

The following list summarizes significant findings in migraine headaches.

1. Usually present in some family member—usually a female member—commonly an aunt, grandmother, mother or sister.

2. Almost always a *one sided* type of headache. May occur at different times on either side, but affects *one entire side of your head;* that is, if you draw an imaginary line through the center of your head dividing the left side of your face from the right, migraine headaches usually involve either the entire right side or the entire left side.

3. Almost always make you sick to your stomach as well as cause a "dilly" of a headache. Vomiting is common.

4. Headache is almost always preceded by an *aura*. Aura means a painless state in which you see wavy lines; have a strange sensation (floating or falling, for instance); or can only see as though you were looking down two tubes (in other words, the visual fields are blocked at the sides, but not in the center).

5. Once migraine starts, both light and noise seem a torture.

6. Almost always found in people who are perfectionists—people who are

extremely conscientious in everything they do and must always do each job flawlessly and in detail lest they feel they have failed.

7. May occur in clusters. That is, you may have a siege of migraines over a period of weeks, then you have none for a long time only to be plagued later again for days or weeks.

HOW JUNE BATTLED HER MIGRAINES

June J., a lady I know who is 30 years old, is married to a rancher in the northwest part of the country. She was city-bred and raised, intelligent, sensitive and a hard worker in everything she did. She never took shortcuts in anything she undertook to do and she was never satisfied with anything less than perfection. All this she carried over with her to her marriage.

June was immediately worried about a lot of things. Will I be a good wife? Will I be a help rather than a hindrance to my husband on the ranch? Can I take being a country girl—alone and isolated—after being used to the city and friends?

All these questions piled up on June and shortly after she moved to the ranch with her new husband, she began having troubles. Of course, June knew she was subject to migraine, but she had them under pretty good control. If she had one or two in a given year, this was about par for the course. But when I next saw her in my office about three months following her marriage, she'd had eight clusters of migraine headaches! And this in spite of the strong medicines she used to try to stop them.

Junes's Program Can Help You with Migraine

The following plan of action enabled June to stop 90 percent of her migraines.

1. June was 30 pounds over ideal weight. She dieted and exercised away the excess.

2. I had June start toning routines just as with anyone losing weight, but I told her to do an extra exercise routine *at the first sign of her aura,* which in her case was seeing small black dots all over her field of vision and a sensation of something dreadful about to happen.

3. Right after her extra exercising, I instructed June to lie flat in bed in a perfectly darkened and noiseless room, and concentrate very strongly on going to sleep and awakening without a headache.

June also found that taking strong black coffee in moderate amounts at the first sign of her aura also helped. Soon, after practice, June found she could reduce the severity of her migraine attack by 50 percent. The attacks which usually lasted all day and all night and sometimes even into the next day, now limited themselves to a few hours—especially, she found, if she could sleep before the excruciating pain started.

I've also noticed over the years that patients have fewer clusters of migraine and the ones that they do have are much less troublesome if they can learn to relax about things they regard as chores. They do better if they can delegate some of their work to others and avoid crowding their schedules every day with many things that can wait until later. In other words, migraine does better when you learn to be less the perfectionist and more the *so what* type of person.

I've already said that migraine is caused by stretching blood vessels. It's the tiny nerve fibers that surround the blood vessels inside your head that are out of whack. They first constrict the vessels (the stage of the aura), then they let go and the vessel suddenly dilates (expands) and this expansion is what brings on all the pain and nausea.

Migraine's Bark Is Much Worse Than Its Bite

You should realize, also, that migraine headaches are perfectly harmless. They do no permanent damage to anything, and they do not pave the way for any dread disease later. But they are devils, as anyone who has had them can tell you. Like June, when you gain better self-control, migraine loses its punch. At present, June no longer takes medicines for migraine—she has found they're not needed. When she does use medicine, it's limited to aspirin and black coffee.

HOW TO EASE SINUS PROBLEMS

The main sinuses are beneath your forehead right above your eyes and directly beneath your cheekbones. The cavities are lined with membranes that secrete mucuous (much like the inside of your mouth). The mucous drains through a tube system into your nose. Anything that plugs up your nose (like a cold) or that blocks off the tubes that lead from the sinuses to your nose (like allergies) can cause a sinus headache.

How to Watch for Sinus Problems

The following table summarizes the typical sinus type headache:

1. Almost always begins in your face. Either above your eyes or beneath your cheeks. If your nose is plugged up, both sets of sinuses can be involved and on both sides of your face. Any one of them may cause trouble by itself.

2. Usually it is the aftermath of a cold with a lot of nose trouble, or it comes on after a siege with allergies (with the usual reaction of swelling, itching, sneezing and so forth).

3. May involve the top of your head or feel like the pain is behind your eyes in the case of the smaller, more deeply seated sinuses.

4. No aura or warning, usually. Usually no nausea or vomiting unless severely infected.

5. More common among persons who have long, thin, narrow noses.

More Sinus Aids Than People

There must be at least a dozen commercial products advertised in newspapers, on TV and elsewhere that go to great lengths to show you what the product does as it goes to work on your sinus headache. The fact is that most do as much harm as good because most of them contain antihistamine drugs. These drugs are drying agents, and it is not the usual state of things for mucous membranes to be completely dried out. To get an idea of what I mean, fill your mouth with cotton and notice the result.

What *is* needed is opening up of the tubes inside your nose that drain the sinuses. These tubes end up on either side of your nose—the cheek side—at about the level of your cheekbone prominence or slightly below it. This means that simply putting drops or sprays inside your nose won't do the job.

YOUR SINUS TREATMENT GUIDE

First, take three aspirin.

Then, lie down flat with your head hanging over the edge or end of the bed or lounge.

Take some plain nose drops—Neosynephrine or Privine will do—and fill up the nostril to the brim on the side where your cheek or forehead aches.

Now turn the affected side down toward the floor, your head still hanging down. Put in another half dropper full of drops. When you do this, you're letting the drops run *into* the affected sinuses where they do their job on the congested membranes.

Now bring your head up on the level, lie with the affected side *up* toward the ceiling, and place a small hot water bottle on the sore area being careful not to burn your skin. Continue the heat for about half an hour—doze off to sleep if you can. Doing this allows the mucous that has gathered in your sinuses to drain out. You may feel the mucous draining down the back of your throat. That's good. It means that your sinuses are at last draining out. When they've finished draining, your pain and discomfort should be gone.

AL'S SUCCESS WITH SINUS CAN ALSO BE YOURS

A patient I know of named Al had chronic sinus trouble and found himself having to go through this procedure more and more often during the winters with repeated colds, flu and so forth. He finally found that he was able to cut down on his sinus headaches about 70 percent by making a habit of sniffing a small amount of salt water into his nose and sinus cavities—using the same position techniques I've already described—once each morning. His method worked with many others I've known and may help you with yours as well.

He dissolved one to one and a half teaspoonsful of ordinary table salt in a pint of warm water, and used about an ounce to an ounce and a half of this solution each time.

HOW TO HANDLE EAR PROBLEMS

Your hearing is one of your most valuable possessions. Any condition that causes a lot of ear infection with "draining ear" problems is potentially a destroyer of hearing later on in life. Therefore, it pays to have your children's painful ears attended to by your medical advisor very early in the game.

How Ear, Sinus, and Nose All Interact with Each Other

Later on in adult life, your ears are affected adversely by other troubles. For example, your inner ear is connected by means of a tiny canal called the Eustachean tube to your throat. This small tube empties out just behind the ones that drain your sinuses. This is why nose troubles can also cause ear troubles. This small canal from your inner ear can get clogged up with air or with mucous from your nose. When it does, trouble can start.

HOW TO KEEP YOUR EARS HEALTHY

1. When you're blowing your nose, leave both sides open—don't close off one side as you may have done in the past. This forces mucous to back up under pressure on the closed side. You run the risk of forcing mucous into your Eustachian tube, thus inviting an ear infection.

2. When you ride a plane or take trips to higher altitudes, make it a habit to yawn and at the same time swallow. This has the affect of keeping your Eustachean tubes unblocked (you may feel this as a *pop* noise in the blocked ear).

3. Inflamed noses, tonsils and adenoids can cause chronic ear problems. This is why you should try to keep plugged up sinuses and noses at least draining during the inflammation—your ears will stay out of trouble if you do.

If your tonsils and adenoids give you more or less intermittent trouble, seek medical advice and have them removed surgically if your advisor agrees. You may be preserving your future hearing capacity by so doing.

LET KEN'S EXPERIENCE HELP YOUR EARS

A man named Ken D. had a recurrent ear blockage problem. Although I couldn't prove it, I believe he had very small Eustachean openings into his throat on one side. The left side of his Eustachean tube would constantly block off and cause Ken to lose a good deal of the hearing in his left ear. Fortunately, Ken did not have too many infections from all this blocking off, otherwise I fear Ken might have lost his hearing almost entirely on this side.

Ear Opening Hints for Your Use

1. Ken bought a nasal bulb at the drug store. This is a small rubber bulb with a snout at one end about an inch or an inch and a half long, tapering at the end to a small opening.

2. Ken squeezed the air from the bulb by simply compressing it with his left hand, then inserted it carefully into his left nasal passage—directing it straight back rather than up or down so that it passed almost all the snout part into his nasal passage.

3. Keeping the bulb compressed all the while, Ken next used a finger to close off the opening to his right nasal passage.

4. Finally, he took a swallow of water into his mouth, held it there to be certain the snout of the bulb was snugly in his left nasal passage and that his right passage was completely closed off.

5. As Ken swallowed the water in his mouth, he released the bulb at the same time, thus making a vacuum in his left nasal passage. This vacuum sucked out the blocked Eustachian tube, thus relieving his condition.

Sometimes Ken had to repeat this several times, but it worked about 90 percent of the time and probably kept his hearing intact. You may also find this maneuver useful for a blocked ear.

The rubber bulb that Ken used is also useful to irrigate your nose and sinuses.

How to Take Care of Your Eardrums

If your eardrum becomes extremely sore and breaks from the pressure built up behind it (draining ear), you need help and should get it as quickly as possible. Your medical advisor will want to put you on antibiotics to stop the infection as rapidly as he can. Once the infection is cleared up, your eardrum should heal and close off shortly thereafter. If it doesn't, the hole needs to be *patched,* a surgical procedure that is very effective and has preserved more hearing than any other procedure I know of.

How to Rid Yourself of Unwanted Wax

The same rubber bulb of which I've spoken is also useful with ear wax problems. It's quite normal for ear canals to secrete wax. Sometimes, an excess occurs and will block your hearing. When this happens, the wax needs to be softened and gently irrigated out of the canal. This can be accomplished most of the time by using hydrogen peroxide (the bubbly liquid that fizzes up when it hits air) dropped into the ear canal, with your head flat on the side opposite the canal you're trying to unblock.

Once you've filled the canal with peroxide from a medicine dropper, you can insert a small cotton plug so it won't all run out. Wait for about half an hour. Then you can fill up the rubber bulb with warm water (not hot) by compressing it and inserting the snout of the bulb into some warm water in your bathroom basin. Insert the snout into the ear canal that's blocked, aim the end of the snout slightly *upward* after you've inserted it about a half to three quarters of an inch into the canal, and then gently and firmly squeeze out the warm water from the bulb. This makes the water flow upwards behind the wax plug and washes it out of your canal.

If the chunk of wax appears at the opening of your ear canal, you can remove it with your fingers or a small pair of tweezers.

Keeping Solid Objects Out of Your Ear Canals

It's obviously very dangerous to insert anything solid into your ear canal. You run the risk of damaging the canal or your eardrum. The rubber snout on the bulb is safe so long as you don't try to push it too far inside the canal, and as long as you squeeze out the water *gently* while the snout is aimed upwardly. Do NOT insert pins, match sticks and so forth inside your ear canals to scrape out wax or other foreign material—let someone do it who can see what he's doing all the while, or use the rubber bulb method.

HOW TO COPE WITH EYE PROBLEMS

Your most important sensory organs are your eyes. Treat them always with the utmost care and respect. Once you lose vision, it may never come back, or it may come back as only a fraction of what it used to be.

How to Handle "Red Eye"

This means anything that causes the whites of your eyes to become bloodshot. The whites of an eye or both eyes get tiny, deep-red vessels on them making them appear red from a distance. This can be caused by almost anything: too much sun, wind, and hot or cold weather; any irritating chemical or fume in the air (smog is a common cause of red eye); too much booze (chronic red eye is almost a tell-tale sign of having a hangover); allergies to pollen, dust or dander in the air (this kind of red eye is almost always accompanied by severe itching, sneezing, and a runny nose as well); and so forth.

If the redness is accompanied as well by eyelids that are stuck shut when you first awaken in the morning, and that matter during the day with a pussy appearing substance, it means that there is infection in your eye as well as irritation, and it should be handled by your medical advisor.

For simple irritation, the most common cause of red eye, all you need to do is to put your eyes at rest for a while—get the irritation away from them. If too much sun is the cause, wear dark colored glasses and stay out of the sun. Eye drops help stop the burn from such irritations and sometimes make them disappear faster. Many of these soothing drops can be found at your druggists and most are safe to use as directed.

An eye wash is also soothing to such eyes. You just fill the eye cup that comes with most of these preparations with the solution, and place it firmly against your closed eye. Tilt your head back, then open your eye so it is bathed in the fluid inside the cup.

If your red eye problem is accompanied by pain—not burning or stinging, but real, honest to goodness pain and/or headaches on that side, you must have your medical advisor check this out. Glaucoma, a disease affecting the inner eye, may start out as a redness particularly around the iris part of the eye; diminished vision; and a headache. It *must* have the help of your advisor for relief.

What to Do About Eye Muscle Problems

When a child or adult looks cross-eyed, he has a squint. The squint may involve only one or both eyes. It means that the muscles that move the eye in a particular direction aren't working just right. Contrary to popular belief, squints generally *do not* go away by themselves, and a child with a squint does *not* outgrow it as a rule.

The trouble with a squint, say in the right eye, is that this eye often becomes lazy in the sense that it doesn't do the job with its share of the vision that it usually does (we all see better from one eye or another, but both are always involved with the seeing we do day in and day out). If this laziness is allowed to continue until the child reaches eight or ten years of age, the lazy eye may lose most if not all of its ability to see as it should. In other words, just like a muscle that's not used, an eye nerve atrophies because it's not used. And it is easily preventable! All children with squints should have glasses whose strong lenses pull the weak eye around so that it sees like the normal one. Failing this, simple corrective surgery can reset the eye muscles so that they work properly.

Do not overlook a young child's squint. His vision may be at stake!

HOW KAREN REGAINED HER VISION

Karen P. was 17 before she realized that her right eye wasn't seeing much of anything. The reason she didn't recognize this was because she'd had a squint since she was quite young, the eye became lazy, and her left eye took over the job of seeing. She didn't realize anything was wrong until one day, quite by accident, she noticed her vision was almost gone with her good left eye shut.

Karen had an eye examination and it was found that her retina (the back of the eye that receives all the visual images) was atrophied, but still healthy. She was a very lucky girl. She had surgery in which one muscle was reset back on her eyeball, and another was reset forward a bit. When it was over, her eye began to see again. Her vision isn't perfect on the right side, but Karen would by now have been totally blind in this eye, without hope of the vision ever returning, had she waited any longer.

How to Tell When Your Vision Needs Attention

In general, it can be said that anything that makes your vision abnormal needs looking in to. And the sooner the better. I would estimate that between hearing problems and vision problems, the two account for more than 90 percent of learning difficulties among children in the lower grades. And if a kid starts off with such a handicap, it will carry over into adult life even though he eventually gets the problem corrected. The point is to always think of eyes and ears whenever your child has difficulties at school—a check on hearing and vision will pay dividends that may well be worth your child's future.

Adults have their particular problems with vision. They have cataracts, glaucoma and farsightedness as the chief offenders. I've already spoken of glaucoma. Cataracts may begin any time, of course, but generally they're a "beyond mid life" situation. They begin by a weakening of vision, especially central vision. In other words, you may see better when you don't look directly at an object than on looking squarely at it. Have this checked, if your eyes behave this way.

Cataracts must be at a certain stage before they can be helped. They must be ripe or it does little good to have them removed. Your medical advisor for eyes is the best judge of this. At the time cataracts must be removed, you can have lenses (contact lenses if you desire) that will compensate for the loss of your eye's lense which is the structure in your eye that cataracts involve.

Farsightedness is noticed when you must hold printed matter or small objects farther and farther away from your eyes in order to see them clearly. This usually happens after age 40 and if you notice this happening to you, you may be farsighted. If it happens, you must have glasses to correct it. The glasses are usually bifocal—the upper part of the lens for normal viewing, the lower for close work. Don't put off getting glasses for this distressing but not serious affliction. Don't let pride interfere with your good vision!

What You Can Do with Eye Injuries

Almost every eye injury can be prevented. Nothing can fly into your eye, for example, if you have goggles or glasses on. Almost every day, I see or hear of someone using a lathe, a grinder, a power saw or other tool without protecting his eyes by putting on goggles. Every day, I see people walk by an area where welding is going on without thinking to glance the other way. Looking at a welder's arc may net you an eye burn. Every day I see children and adults looking right into the bright sun—a good way to burn a hole in your retina! When observing an eclipse of the sun, use a strong filter between the sun and your eyes, like X-ray film or heavily smoked glass. Better still, reflect the eclipse on a piece of paper, looking away from the sun entirely. You'll protect your eyes from damage if you do.

If you ever have reason to suspect something has flown into your eye, *always* have it checked by your medical advisor. Even if you can't see or feel anything in your eye at the time, have it checked. Small metal or wooden pieces—the size of a grain of sand or smaller—can actually perforate your eyeball and cause irreparable damage inside your eye, and you can neither see nor feel it in there at first!

The most common injury is a small foreign object—a speck of dust or whatever—getting stuck beneath your upper eyelid. When this happens, every time you blink you feel a scratchy sensation in your eye; it gets red and waters, and tears flow.

YOUR GUIDE TO CINDER REMOVAL

When you look inside someone's eye for something in it, the following methods will help you and the person with the trouble.

1. Have him lay down flat in a darkened room. Ask him to look straight up toward the ceiling of the room. Use a flashlight with fresh batteries.

2. Carefully look beneath his lower eyelid by simply pulling downwardly on the skin beneath the lower lid. You can see inside the sac thus produced very easily. If something's in there, you'll see it.

3. Next, ask him to look down toward his feet and keep his eyes directed there. Grasp his upper eyelid lashes with your left hand while at the same time *gently* depressing the skin of his upper lid downwardly. This (with a little practice) has the effect of turning his upper eyelid inside out—the inner surface of his upper eye lid is pooched out, and if you keep his lashes held against the upper part of his eyelid, it will stay that way while you scan his inner upper eyelid for any foreign objects.

4. If you find something, take a thin wisp of cotton and try to dislodge and lift it up. If this fails, run some water over it from a small glass or eye cup. This will usually wash it out into the eye, where his blinking will cause it to lodge in one of the two corners of his eye. Then you can remove it with your fingers—*gently*!

If this fails, or if you see something stuck in the center clear bulge of his eye (his cornea) don't try any further maneuvers, but ask for help from your medical advisor.

Putting the Injured Eye at Rest

In general, any eye injury that hurts and is worse when the eye is blinking or moving around had best be patched shut while some professional help is sought. To do this, simply place a cotton ball (or two) gently over the closed eye, tear off several strips of half inch tape or scotch tape and lay them over the cotton ball, and attach the strips to his forehead and cheek. Lay several such strips overlapping each other so that when you're through, he should be able to open his good eye and see no light from the patched one.

Don't Make Laura's Mistake

Be leery of black eyes. Usually they're harmless, but they can spell trouble. I know a young Midwestern farm mother named Laura F. for example, who was out in the backyard playing with her young kids. She was the catcher, her young son was batting. Her other son pitched the ball; the batting son swung, missed the ball, but caught Laura square in her left eye. In minutes, Laura had a real shiner—the skin around her left eye was black and blue and the whites of her eye reddened. Her husband chided her for being too close to the bat when he got home later on.

The next morning, Laura noticed she saw double from her left eye—when she put her hand over her right eye, the left eye saw two of everything. X rays later that day revealed Laura had a blow-out fracture of the orbit—a crack in the bony case that surrounds the eyeball. She needed extensive surgery to correct the damage. So the rule of thumb is, don't neglect to get help with a black eye any time you notice vision troubles following a black eye, from whatever cause.

WHAT YOU CAN DO ABOUT NOSE PROBLEMS

Broken noses are rather common. You get hit in the nose with a baseball, the dashboard of the car, the human hand or whatever. Later, your nose swells up and you can't breathe too well through your nose. In addition, there is bruising over the bridge of your nose. These signs indicate that your rather frail nose bones have been cracked.

THE CRITICAL QUESTIONS TO ASK ABOUT NOSE INJURIES

1. Is the bleeding stopped or does it continue? (There is always some degree of nosebleed following most blows to the nose—more if there is an injury to the bones.)
2. Is your nose line—the middle front ridge of your nose from its start at your forehead to its termination at the tip of your nose—to the right or left of the midline?
3. Look at the injured nose from the bottom. (Have the injured party tilt his head backward or you do the same in front of a mirror). Does the piece of your nose that runs across the bottom, dividing the nose into two compartments run straight, or does it curve, or is it shoved upward?

If the answer to any of these questions is yes, chances are good that your nose has suffered injury that needs repair. For this, your medical advisor should be sought.

Handling Long Nasal Hairs

One of the most common mistakes I see people making regarding their noses is in pulling out long nasal hairs that sometimes stick out the nasal passage. These hairs are imbedded in very sensitive mucous membranes just inside your nose and if you use force to pull them out, you stand a good chance of starting an infection at the base of the hair.

The way to handle long nasal hairs is simply to trim them off flush with the nostril with sharp scissors, or a razor blade or electric shaver. Don't pull them out.

Nosebleeds

A bleeding nose is common and all sorts of things have been devised to stop them. It's one thing to get them stopped, another to deal with the condition that causes it. Bleeding from a nose is usually from the partition down the center of your nose that divides it into separate cavities. This partition is made of gristle and has a rich network of very small arteries and veins imbedded in it. The vessels in the front lower third of this partition are the ones that do 98 percent of the bleeding.

HOW TO STOP MOST NOSEBLEEDS

1. Sit up, your head tilted slightly forward.
2. Pinch together your nostrils such that the pressure of such pinch is directly against the middle partition of your nose. Breathe entirely through your mouth.
3. Hold firm constant pressure in this manner for no less than 15 minutes. Sometimes it takes half an hour.

It is of no avail to apply ice packs to your neck or forehead or to go through all sorts of gyrations and contortions with nosebleeds. Pressure is what does the trick. And the pressure has to be directly on the bleeding vessels. Once in a while, bleeding will come from far back in your nose where you can't possibly get to it. This will require help from your medical advisor to stop.

Dry weather, cold weather, and allergic troubles all predispose one to nosebleeds. Any time your nose is struck, it may bleed. Picking or blowing your nose too hard will also cause bleeding.

Dry membranes in the nose are easily corrected—just paint the dry membranes with mineral oil or glycerin on a cotton swab, two or three times a day, especially before you have to go out in the cold or dry weather. This will keep the membranes moist and stop the bleeding tendency.

HOW MEL'S NOSEBLEED WAS STOPPED

I recall a man named Mel M. who tried all these things with a particularly severe nosebleed one day and nothing worked. It was really bleeding profusely. He'd never had any such thing before and was in good health otherwise.

When I looked in Mel's nose with a light and using a suction apparatus so I could see what was going on, I found a little tiny pumping artery on the wall opposite the partition of Mel's nose. In order to stop this tiny pumper (arteries pump, veins ooze) I had to use an electric cautery. This is an instrument that makes a small electric spark that coagulates the tissue it hits. Sometimes this is the only way to stop a stubbornly bleeding nose.

SUMMARY

1. You can deal with most headaches with no more than aspirin, strong coffee and rest. Other headaches are rare and can be recognized by following the rules for serious headaches.
2. Your nose, sinus cavities and ears are all interwoven as far as the good health of each is concerned. If you follow principles of good health with all three, you'll have far less trouble with any single area.
3. Your eyes are extremely important to you. Take meticulous care of red eye, infections, injuries, and visual problems early and swiftly in order to prevent serious, permanent damage.
4. If bleeding from your nose doesn't stop in a reasonable time, seek professional help. If an injury to your nose occurs, look first at the contour to judge whether you need help.

HOW TO PUT STRENGTH AND ZIP INTO AILING MUSCLE AND BONE   163

treatment of each form in spite of all the new drugs and hormones and in spite of the current fads brought forth for treatment. Your medical advisor should decide on any stronger treatment.
4. Care of the feet requires the sensible use of moleskin, or felt padding with adhesive on one side; soakings; and good sense with shoes and the treatment of any infection.

12

How to Apply Common Sense Health to Menstrual and Menopausal Difficulties

There are menstrual difficulties that seem forever to plague women. You'll discover how to handle them in this section. Along with menstrual problems are the common questions and problems concerned with "the pill" and with the IUD (Intrauterine device) for preventing pregnancy. Such problems are vital and need to be discussed, and we'll talk about these questions in this section.

The menopause is always an interesting time of life—both men and women have all sorts of problems supposedly based on menopause and its effects. These problems will be elaborated on in relation to both sexes and we will see what you can do about them.

Finally, there are some long standing myths about how menopause affects general health. These myths will be exposed and you'll discover how it's possible to remain perfectly well and healthy during this time—perhaps even better than previously!

HOW TO COME TO TERMS WITH MENSTRUATION

In talking with thousands of women, I've found that the best attitude toward menstruating every month comes from those who view it with the least resentment, as the least chore, and with the fewest fears. This may sound strange, but its true.

Virtually 99 percent of the problems with menstruation are preconditioned—that is, they're planted by someone else in the minds of young women and there they stick. There are of course, unusual causes for menstrual difficulties, but they are rare. Mostly it's just a habit—a way of looking at something as natural as day and night.

Menstruation occurs in cycles. Each woman's cycle is, for her, uniquely her own. No two women have quite the same cycle, but they're similar in many ways. The reason for the cycle is built into the female hormone balance since it's entirely owing to hormones that menstruation occurs. Simply stated, the first phase of the cycle begins with the first day of bleeding (menstruation); phase two begins on the day bleeding stops and includes the day the egg pops out of one of the ovaries; and phase three is the interval between this time and the first day of bleeding—the complete cycle.

Phase one begins because a special hormone has built up the lining inside the uterus in preparation for a fertilized egg from the ovary. When an unfertilized egg is presented, this hormone production is stopped, the lining of the uterus is sloughed off, and menstruation begins. After menstruation stops, the build-up of a second hormone occurs that is the basis for the next cycle. At about mid-point (10-14 days) into phase two, ovulation occurs and the cycle is repeated again.

Probably one of the most common of menstrual complaints is that of menstrual cramps. Usually they begin just before phase one, and may continue for one or more days. I cannot count the number of women I've seen who "just can't stand" these cramps and many of them actually must go to bed because of them.

HOW PENNY CONTROLLED MENSTRUAL CRAMPS

Penny R., a young lady of 23, was one such person. She thought something was wrong her cramps were so bad. After examining her, I found nothing wrong, so I began to talk with Penny about her background. I found that she had been raised to view the menstrual process as "a horrible ordeal, messy, and a blight on the female of the species." I further learned that Penny had normal periods for the first couple of years. It wasn't until she reached her late teens that her cramps began to get her down.

Penny's Program for Easier Periods

Here is the routine Penny found stopped her cramps. You may find it helpful as well.

1. Penny was only a few pounds overweight, but was sadly soft and out of physical condition. She started toning routines in the morning and at night.

2. The week before her periods were to start, I had her *increase* her physical activity. Yes, increase it! I had her do bicycle riding, swimming and/or hiking in addition to her toning routines.

It may go without saying that Penny didn't like this a bit. She found it enough of a chore just to start physical toning, let alone all this "athletic bit," as she put it. I did manage to convince her to at least try it for a couple of periods—if nothing happened, she could quit.

3. The week before her periods, I also had Penny go on a strictly salt-free diet. And I mean strict. No salt in cooking or added to foods or any prepared food with salt in it. I asked her to restrict her fluid intake by about a third—not allow herself to become unduly thirsty, just to cut down one glass out of every three of her daily fluids—*just for the five to seven days before her period was to begin.*

4. For any distress she felt in her pelvic region, I limited her medicine to aspirin (or tylenol—an aspirin like drug), in doses of two or three every three or four hours as needed, and nothing else.

Penny found that after only two months of this schedule, she had her period cramps under such control that going to bed because of them was no longer necessary. In fact, Penny discovered that contrary to her own belief in this matter, the more physical activity she did during the week preceding her period, the better she felt and the fewer cramps she had!

HOW EXCESS BLEEDING CAN BE CONTROLLED

Periods usually establish themselves pretty well as to how much bleeding and how long they last, on the average. Some women normally bleed only a day and a half or two, and very lightly at that; others bleed for the greater part of a week and taper off only after ten days. If the pattern has established itself, it may vary a little, but not much from month to month.

There are a number of things that can affect the bleeding patterns of menstruation. Most are harmless and require nothing more than careful observation on your part. If you've been used to having four or five day periods, for example, and suddenly they start going good for ten or twelve days, something is wrong.

Lori's Unusual Case

The last lady I saw with this kind of alteration in menstrual bleeding was Lori H., a lady of 37 years, mother of three, and previously healthy. She had put on weight steadily over the past couple of years and she noticed that she tired quite easily doing things she used to breeze through before.

In checking Lori, it was discovered she had developed an underactive thyroid gland—the gland in your neck that controls your body's metabolism (the rate your cells burn up energy).

When this was corrected, Lori's periods returned to normal and she has remained well since.

When You Should View Bleeding with Suspicion

When there is bleeding from your vaginal canal at any other time than what is usual for your period, it must be viewed with suspicion. For example, if you notice bleeding after intercourse (normal for newlyweds, but not after you've been married a couple of years, and certainly *not* after menopause), between periods, or after physical exertion, this needs the attention of your medical advisor. He'll want to do the routine "Pap smears" and a pelvic examination to get at the cause. These types of abnormal bleeding should *not* be put off, but should be brought to someone's attention *promptly* so that they may be stopped.

One word of consideration for you women with vaginal bleeding problems: It's quite possible for you to have blood passing from either your urethra (the tube leading from your bladder to the outside) or from your rectum. In both cases such bleeding may appear to be coming, or you may just naturally attribute it to coming, from your vagina. To check this, insert a tampon type napkin into your vagina, and observe the toilet paper and the character of your stools after you empty your bowels and after you've urinated. If one of these two other places is the cause of the bleeding, it will become apparent.

SOME IDEAS ABOUT "THE PILL" THAT WILL HELP YOU

In this day and age we've all heard and read much about "the pill" and its uses as a contraceptive (prevention of pregnancy). We've been able to observe the effects of the pill now for about six or seven years—enough to give a pretty good idea of how it works, what you can expect and not expect of it, and what the advantages and disadvantages are.

The following list summarizes the effects of the pill.

1. It's quite effective in preventing pregnancies (nothing is 100 percent effective). If you take them strictly as directed, you won't have to worry about becoming pregnant.

2. A small percentage of side effects are seen. The most common one I've seen is a tendency to become mentally depressed while on them. Another is a tendency to put on weight (largely in the form of retained water from the affects of the hormones in the pill).

3. The pill does not prolong or put off menopause nor does it cause you to stay "available for being pregnant" long after you would normally become infertile as a natural course of events. (Anytime after 42 or 43 years of age in women.)

4. Sometimes "breakthrough bleeding" will occur while you're taking the pill. Breakthrough bleeding means that during the three week cycle of the month that you take the pill, you may begin to bleed slightly though you're not supposed to do any bleeding until you stop taking them during the fourth week of the month. This is not serious nor is it hazardous in the sense that you're suddenly likely to become pregnant. It's just a nuisance usually managed by ignoring it entirely.

Blood Clotting Trouble

There was much talk at first about the pill causing blood clotting disturbances. In the hundreds of women I've seen on this drug, I've only seen one lady who had this trouble. I think that in her case it was definitely caused from the pill, but she recovered rapidly from the trouble and enjoys good health today. If it does occur, it means no more taking the pill from that point on. The likelihood of this complication, in my opinion, is rare.

One Bonus of the Pill that You May Look Forward to

Of course, an obvious advantage of the pill used in this way for contraceptive reasons is that if you happen to have irregular or unreliable menstrual periods to begin with, use of the pill will automatically straighten them out. The reason for this is that the hormones in the pill prevent ovulation, and they control when your period comes—phase one starts within a day or two of discontinuing the pill, and stops within a day or two after starting to take the pill again.

The pill does not affect your sexual ability as a woman. In fact, if anything, the release from the mental worry of becoming pregnant when you don't want to is usually a stimulus to enjoying sex more than before.

HOW THE IUD MAY BENEFIT YOU

The other partner in the duet of modern contraception is the

IUD (abbreviation for Intrauterine Device) so called because it is a small plastic and/or metal device that is inserted inside the uterine cavity. In this location it prevents pregnancy from occurring though exactly why no one really knows. The point is, it works. And it does so without any of the drawbacks of having to take drugs. The following list summarizes the status of the IUD.

1. There can be no systemic effects such as are bound to occur when you are taking drugs.
2. There is no having to remember to take a pill or shot.
3. The insertion of an IUD is not difficult and only slightly uncomfortable.
4. There are some women who have bleeding problems with an IUD inserted. These problems are generally mild and stop of their own accord. They sometimes upset the usual menstrual period patterns.

An IUD is inserted in the doctor's office. Attached to the ends of the device are two small "strings" which are allowed to remain where they can be reached when it is desired to remove the device.

Which One for You?

I usually recommend that young, newly married women use the pill for the first year or two of their marriage. After this time or any time after their first child, if they have one, I recommend use of the IUD from then on. I find this routine is far more effective, much better tolerated in the long run, and the most effective combination of contraception.

I think the ideal contraceptive has yet to be invented, but I think it is only a matter of a short time until it is.

HOW TO DEAL WITH MENOPAUSE

I suppose of all the misinformation and misgiving among women, menopause has taken the number one spot. Is menopause really all that bad? Is it the devastating, deflorating monster it's claimed to be? Must you stop living because of menopause? No, of course not. In fact, you can begin to really live after menopause.

HOW MARLENE REACTED TO MENOPAUSE

Marlene K. was 46, and lived in a rural village. For the past eight months her periods had been diminishing and getting scantier. Finally they'd stopped. Marlene was panic stricken—not because she didn't know what was happening, but because of the fear of what was going to happen.

She appeared in my office one day, the picture of dejectedness. The world seemed about to come to an end. When I asked her what in thunder it was that had gotten her down, she looked down at the floor and whispered in almost inaudible tones that she had just reached menopause and would I do whatever it was that doctors are supposed to do to help.

I was flabbergasted! For awhile I didn't know exactly what to say to this intelligent women—the wife and mother in a happy, prosperous family and with virtually everything to look forward to. Finally I answered, "What exactly do you want me to do?" She slowly looked up at me, surprised, and a little angry, and replied, "Why, start the hormones, of course. And the tonics and vitamins!"

Marlene's comment is the same as I've heard from far too many women in menopause. I explained to Marlene that in the first place, hormones aren't used routinely, at least I don't use them. Why? Because usually the aren't needed. There are only two signs that hormones help with, I told Marlene. And, although not rare, neither are they common.

The first of these is hot flashes. Hot flashes occur usually during the first few months of menopause in *some* women. They are felt as sudden, intense, warm flushes all over the body, usually accompanied also by nervousness, jitteriness and depression. They are generally short-lived and will disappear by themselves even if no therapy is given. If hot flashes become a nuisance, then taking estrogen will help. Estrogen is given by mouth in small, even doses every day for a few weeks to a couple of months. Then it is discontinued.

If the flashes return, the estrogen can be started again for a short time. Estrogen *never needs to be given by injection,* as I've heard many women say that is the advice they've received. In the first place, hormone shots are expensive, and in the second, their levels in the system can't possibly be controlled when given by a shot. The most important reason for not giving hormone shots is simply that they are not needed—taking estrogen by mouth is quite enough.

Another Indication for Hormones

The second and only other sign that indicates hormones are

necessary is the drying out of the vaginal mucous membranes that sometimes occurs for a short time early in menopause.

The menopause is, of course, characterized by the diminuation of your natural estrogen levels. Estrogen is primarily produced in your ovaries. Menopause shuts your ovaries down, and so there is less estrogen. Notice that I didn't say shuts them *off*—just diminshes their activity. It is true that menopause does shut off ovulation (the shedding of an egg every month as during phase two of menstruation), but you still have some estrogen—enough to meet your needs the rest of your life.

When the estrogen levels are diminished, sometimes the effect on the normally moist mucous membranes in your vaginal tracts is to dry them somewhat. If this occurs, it will be only temporary and can be corrected for the short time it lasts by using one of several available estrogen cremes that you can apply once or twice a day with an applicator or with your fingers. This will stop the drying effect.

WHY NAOMI'S SEXUAL FEARS WERE GROUNDLESS

Another woman I know, named Naomi F., was 50 years old when her menopause occurred. She came to me in tears and when I finally found out the real cause of her concern, she told me she was worried sick. Her husband, it seemed, was a sexually vigorous man and since she was about to lose her sexual capacity with the oncoming of menopause, she supposed he'd either leave her, or perhaps seek out other company.

This is another myth of menopause. If anything, sexual capacity is increased! The reason for this is so simple: No longer is there fear of pregnancy and no longer is there need for contraceptives. Both these reasons bring about a much more relaxed and interested atmosphere regarding sex so that there is actually renewed zest with sex.

Menopause has absolutely nothing to do with sexual desire except that the increasing age of your body normally brings about some reduction in sex desire over the years.

As it happened in Naomi's case, she conceded to me after a couple of sessions in which she was able to discuss the problem calmly that she was never highly interested in sex even when in her twenties. What she actually feared was that it would all disappear and that she might drive her husband elsewhere. Time soothed Naomi's fears and showed her how unnecessary they really were.

How to Snap Out of Menopausal Blues

There is no doubt that menopause brings with it some temporary sinking of the spirits. This is mental, not physical, and may be tied up with many other problems in a woman's life that have nothing whatsoever to do with sex, hormone levels, or aging. Usually, these problems were previously there. Now, with the lessening of womanly attributes such as menstruation, family responsibilities (at least with the raising of youngsters), and so on, she has nothing else to hang on to, or so she believes. A blue mood results.

OPAL'S METHOD OF DEALING WITH MENOPAUSAL BLUES

Opal Z. was such a person. When it became obvious that her depression was the overriding symptom of her menopause at age 51, I told her that she could overcome it without having to go to a psychiatrist to undergo analysis or any such thing. All she had to do was to adhere to the following schedule:

1. Reduce weight. Opal was **45** pounds overweight—a rather common finding among menopausal women, especially those who are depressed, I've noticed.
2. Start vigorous toning routines. I worked Opal up to 30 minutes three times a day—more than she needed, but with depression, more physical exercise hastens its disappearance.
3. Stop secluding herself; stop feeling sorry for herself; and let others help her through this trial. Her husband was helpful. He took her out more often, sometimes even when Opal didn't really want to go out. He also saw to it that their children (grown) made it a point to present minor problems for Opal to solve—made her feel wanted and needed.
4. Increase her intake of coffee, tea and cola drinks during the day to take advantage of the mild stimulation of the caffeine in them. But drink none of these at supper time or thereafter, however, so as to insure proper sleep.
5. Stop the hormone shots she was taking. She thought they were necessary—had convinced herself they were—but learned much to her surprise that not only weren't they needed, but that she also felt better when she stopped them!
6. Involve her mind. Get interested in anything that would force her to think or use her mind. In Opal's case, one of the best things she did in this

regard was to become involved in her county political party's election caucuses. She also became interested in political history and became an expert on the subject by extensive reading.

To sum it all up about menopause: It is, indeed, the start of the golden years because you are set free. You can do what you want because you have more time; you can enjoy life because you appreciate it more; and you can grow physically and mentally by applying principles of common sense health!

WHAT TO DO ABOUT MALE MENOPAUSE

Think a minute. Haven't you read or known men beyond 60 years of age becoming fathers? It's not at all uncommon. Have you ever heard of a woman becoming a mother beyond 60? I never have. Men don't have the same definite period of menopause in their lives as women do.

Art's Fears of Menopause

I once talked to a man named Art E. who was 57 years old. He was being treated for gonorrhea. When I asked him why he was seeking female companionship since he was happily married to a very attractive woman, he replied, "Well, I'll be getting impotent one of these days, and I'd better get in all I can before it happens." When I asked him why he thought he'd be impotent, he said, "I figure I'm on borrowed time now. Should have gone through the change a long time ago."

To be sure, men do show a gradual slowing throughout their lives in interest and in frequency of sex contact. A man can't be as active at 60 as he was at 20, for instance. This is just the slowing down that's inevitable in everyone, not the onset of male menopause.

Adam's Request for Menopause Hormones

Another man I know named, Adam M., came to me with a flat request for male hormones. It seems he was 45. Wasn't he going to need them soon? Especially to satisfy his wife who was 15 years his junior? No, I told him, he wouldn't. I tell men in their 60's and 70's the same thing when they marry a young woman rather late in life.

The plain fact is, giving male hormones to an elderly man will do nothing for his sex capacity and only serve to make his prostate larger and cause more trouble than anything he had before he started taking hormones.

What men should realize before late marriages is that no one, including a young wife, should expect him to perform sexually just as if he were 25 years old. It simply isn't in the books. Another plain fact is that most 25 or 30 year old women who marry 65 or 70 year old men don't expect it. If they do, either they are dreadfully naive or simply foolish. Most marriages at such ages aren't made for sexual pleasure, though older people do indeed have sexual enjoyment, but at a much slower pace than when they were younger. Sexual contact at 70 may be once every month or eight weeks—or even four or five times a year.

HOW YOU CAN ACHIEVE LASTING HEALTH
DURING MENOPAUSE

There is absolutely no reason why you can't continue going right at top efficiency during and following menopause. There may be some adjustments in your program for health at this time, but they are easily made.

Keeping up Your Physical Condition

Now it's even more important to do daily toning routines. Why? Because you tend to get a little lazy about menopause time—your life may slow down a bit, you may eat a little more, and you may not get the normal exercise every day you used to. This makes it important to *increase your efforts* in this area!

Put Your Nutrition on a High Plane and Keep It There

After menopause, you may notice a decided tendency to put on weight more rapidly. Part of this is from the hormone decrease, part of it because it's easier to eat than to occupy your mind and body with activities that require exertion. That is all the more reason to embark on health control at this time or to increase your efforts if you already take good care of your body.

Remember that even if you have to have surgery around this time, when you recover sufficiently to become active, this is the time to start toning and diet to bring weight and muscle tone to optimum levels. Don't postpone it. Don't let yourself slip into habits of too much lounging around on your backside, and too much rich food. Start today with that diet and those exercises. You'll be glad you did!

Are There "Menopausal Diseases"?

There are no diseases that are more apt to plague you during or after menopause than before, *if you're taking care of your health properly*. Having already started health control, you've taken a giant step toward sustained good health. You've already taken steps that will head off heart, blood vessel, and arthritic disease, for example. And you're increasing your lung power and keeping your digestive system working at top efficiency. Keep at it! You'll never have cause to regret it!

SUMMARY

1. You can easily overcome most menstrual difficulties by utilizing the rules of health control and by considering the phases of your cycle during which trouble may occur.
2. The pill and the IUD are the two modern contraceptive devices that are effective. They are preferable to any one of the ones used before they came along. They are an integral part of health control before menopause.
3. Menopause is much overdone as a cause for ills. Your health should actually improve after menopause. Men do not have menopause as such.

13

How to Deal with Common
and Uncommon Infections

We'll discuss the common cold in this section. You'll discover how you can prevent the majority of them and what to do when you do get one.

The flu is now blamed for all sorts of ails and aches. True influenza is a serious disease and most people who have the flu don't really have influenza at all. You'll learn how to tell the flu from a host of other things and what to do with it if it should occur.

Next in common order are skin infections. Most of these, too, can be prevented if not kept in check. Once in a while a skin infection will get out of hand. You should know what to do if and when it does.

The common streptococcus (strep, for short) is a real pain. You should know how to recognize it and what to do about it. Blood vessel infections are another source of much confusion. We'll talk about what to do when one of these infections develop.

HOW TO DEAL WITH COLDS

Every year, millions of people are afflicted with the common cold. Colds can range from a mild nasal sniffle for a couple of days to general aches, pains, feeling like the very devil, mild fever, plugged up sinuses, stuffy nose, watery eyes and congested chest.

Colds, or better, the cold syndrome, are supposed to be caused by viruses. There are at least three dozen different strains of viruses that have been incriminated as causing colds. Still, we're no better treating colds now than a hundred years ago. Why should this be? I'd like to offer the following case history as one reason—perhaps a main reason—why it is that colds have eluded the scientific approach for so long.

You May Find Clem's Experience Helpful with Your Colds

Clem W. was a young man, married and with three children. He was high strung, easily upset and had a job with a co-op firm that kept him on edge.

When I first began to see Clem as a patient, most of his complaints revolved around vague aches and pains that were obviously caused from his reacting to almost everything and anything as though they all were crises. Everything was at the edge of disaster, or at least that's the way Clem looked at it. I also noticed that Clem had one cold after another, both winter and summer; and he wasn't allergic to anything that we could find.

Over the first few years I came to know Clem, these colds became worse—he had more of them, and they hit him with more severity each year, it seemed. And they were beginning to get him down, literally as well as figuratively.

I puzzled over Clem's predicament. Why should he have so many colds? He was healthy as a horse, young, vigorous and robust. After long thought and analysis of past records, I came to a conclusion that since has proven itself hundreds of times in as many patients: Clem's problem with colds was based on emotional upheavals!

That's right! I said emotions. How could this be? How could any mental state affect the body? I don't think we have all the answers to this question, but when I began to attack Clem's problem (and subsequently many others) with this in mind, he got better! And without any miracle drugs, antibiotics or unctions—all of which Clem had tried in the past without results.

FIVE STEPS TO HELP PREVENT COLDS

The following program brought about the best control of recurrent colds in Clem's case and in hundreds of other cases as well.

1. I sat down and had a long talk with Clem about what I thought was producing so much of his cold troubles. I was frank to admit that it probably wasn't the only problem—the only cause for his colds—but perhaps a major one. He at least agreed to try a new approach.

2. First, I had Clem learn several relaxing approaches—how and when to make his mind settle down in spite of the "crucial crisis" of the moment. It was difficult. Clem wasn't used to taking things easily or lightly. If worse

came to worse, I told him, I wanted him to *avoid* any situations at work or at home that might precipitate an emotional upheaval—a crisis.

3. Next, I had him promise to do one thing when he felt an acute case of nerves coming on in spite of his efforts to avoid it: He was to spend the next 20 or 30 minutes, regardless of where he might be at the time, with some type of *exertive physical activity*. It might be punching a bag; a two or three mile jog; a swim in a pool, if one were handy; chopping a cord of wood—anything that would really work up a head of steam.

4. Next, I asked Clem about his family circumstances. Was there any trouble with his spouse, with the kids, or with anything in the household that brought on crises? Yes, he said, there were a number of things, and he went on to enumerate arguments with his wife about who should control the money; about whose feelings should come first, his wife's or his or the kids'; about discipline problems; and so on. I asked him to work these out, slowly and thoroughly, so that things would go smoothly in the home.

5. I asked Clem to cut his smoking to five cigarettes or less a day. He happened to be a heavy smoker (two to three packs a day) and many of his numerous colds went "down to his chest."

You can think what you want about this problem of emotional stress in the production of colds—I'm frank to admit that fifteen years ago, or even ten, I'd have laughed at the absurdity of the thing. But it works!

Within six months, Clem noticed a decided decrease not only in the number of colds he had, but in their severity as well. After a year and a half, Clem cut down his cold frequency to about three a year (from a previous high of ten or twelve). Five years later, Clem felt put upon if he had one cold a year!

I've seen this work in a variety of circumstances, and in a variety of patients with good health, but who had a lot of colds every year, year in and year out. In young, old, and middle-aged people, in men and women of all races, creeds and colors. So it seems to me perfectly justifiable to hang the blame of the common cold—in the main—to disturbing emotional upsets that affect different people in different ways.

To test the theory yourself, begin to make a mental if not written record of your own colds. Note in particular when they start and see if you don't find an emotional ruffling in the picture somewhere. I don't say that we should all try to be unemotional robots—this is impractical and undesirable. What I'm saying is that if we can learn to avoid getting *upset* and *disturbed* for long periods of time with the ups and downs of life, we can probably cut down the incidence of the common cold 80 percent or more!

The Abuse of Antibiotics in Colds

Unfortunately, in many respects, we are a nation of drug users. These days, it's considered either inhuman or unethical to say anything against the use of drugs. In my opinion, Americans take too many drugs for their own good. Some drugs, of course, are necessary to continuing good health, but they are definitely overused.

Antibiotics are among the overused kind. When penicillin was discovered back in the early 40's, it was the first "miracle" type drug. Penicillin was used to treat almost everything that could possibly be termed an infection, and innumerable conditions other than infections. When indicated for a group of certain infections, penicillin is quite effective—or was until two things happened:

1. Many people had so much of it they became allergic to it and could no longer take it.
2. It was used so much that it lost its power to kill some strains of germs for which it was once effective.

No one can help it if they develop an allergy to medicine. It seems the more effective and potent a drug is, the more apt it is to cause bad reactions in the systems of more and more people.

However, it can be helped if the drug is used so much it loses its punch. The most overused side of penicillin was and still is in giving it to people with the common cold and flu. Penicillin—and for that matter any other antibiotic—is NOT effective against colds and flu. It should not be used. Antibiotics cannot kill viruses. Often, in fact, the virus increases in power in the presence of antibiotics.

HOW TO DECIDE IF ANTIBIOTICS ARE NEEDED

1. If a bacterial infection adds itself to a cold or flu. Antibiotics will then help kill off the germs. They will NOT alter the progress of the cold or flu virus.
2. If an individual who is in delicate health to begin with gets a cold or

flu—has a severe heart or lung condition, for example—antibiotics may sometimes be helpful in preventing such people from becoming seriously ill with their colds or flu.

Ida's Experience

A lady named Ida K. that I know was used to having penicillin with every sniffle. Nothing you could tell this lady or explain to her would shake her from the firm belief that penicillin cured her colds.

Ida came to me one day with a minor cold. She demanded penicillin. When I refused after making sure the cold was all that was going on, she became quite irate. I lost her as a patient.

She went to another doctor who gladly gave her penicillin. She had developed an allergy to penicillin over the years, unbeknownst to her, and this shot was the one that really broke the camel's back, so to speak. Ida had an acute anaphylactic shock condition from the penicillin—that is, she reacted violently to it and her breathing apparatus was involved to such an extent that she stopped breathing rather suddenly.

Ida recovered after a stormy period in which she had to have cortisone and artificial breathing. A rather heavy price to pay, though, for not being willing to listen to sound advice.

HOW TO COPE WITH THE FLU

Fortunately, of all the viruses that make the rounds from October to March most are not true influenza. The "flu" (non-influenza viruses) does make people ill—however, not as ill as real influenza.

A Typical Flu Case

Boris G. had an episode of one of these flu viruses last winter. His case is typical so I'll relate it here. Boris first noticed he felt lousy when he arose from a good night's sleep. He just didn't feel right though he couldn't put his finger on anything that hurt or bothered. His energy level was low and he had to force himself to move. He ate breakfast and went to work. He continued to feel weak and out of it.

By mid afternoon, Boris felt feverish and flushed and had the sensation of chilling now and again. By evening, on returning home from work, Boris noticed his back muscles ached. He didn't eat dinner, but went right to bed.

The next morning, Boris noticed headache and a burning sensation inside his nose and cheekbone area. His weakness had progressed to the point of incapacitation. He was relieved by using aspirin.

The next day, Boris noticed canker sores (cold sores or fever blisters) inside his mouth and nose. With the appearance of this new sign, his weakness, fatigue, loss of appetite, and aching back muscles stopped. The sores persisted about a week, then disappeared.

This case is typical of a lot I see every winter. It's caused by a virus known as *Herpes virus*. It's the same one that causes just cold sores without the rest of the flu-like symptoms, especially among women. It's also related to both the chicken pox virus and the one that causes shingles.

How to Treat the Flu

Treatment in this case, as with most such viruses, is limited to *bed rest* (an important part of therapy not taken into consideration by large numbers of people), plenty of fluids, and large doses of aspirin. If there is a cough—caused by the virus getting into your chest and irritating your breathing tubes—you can get relief by using any of a number of cough medicines on your druggist's shelf. They don't cure the cough—they just modify it enough so that it isn't the aggravation it usually is.

It's perfectly true that complications can occasionally set in with any virus or flu bug. The following rules of thumb will help you tell when this happens:

1. Fever is not unusual during the first stages of flu. It doesn't generally persist very long. If the original fever (between 100 and 102 degress) comes down to normal, but later spikes up again, suspect complications and seek medical advice.

2. If your breathing tree becomes very congested with difficulty in taking a breath any time after flu starts, have this checked, especially if accompanied by a heavy phlegm that takes on a green-yellow or blood tinged appearance.

3. If severe headache follows any virus infection and is accompanied by drowsiness, stupor, or "out of head" talk, seek immediate help from your medical advisor.

Proper Use of Flu Vaccine

For the common strains of true influenza, there are good vaccines available. To be effective, such vaccines should be taken beginning in October with a booster in December or January. At present, only people who are ill from chronic diseases are advised to take such vaccines routinely every year, unless an epidemic is expected. This is gauged by the Public Health Service on the basis of information gathered from around the world. They are generally accurate in their predictions.

A USEFUL LIST OF FLU PREDISPOSING AGENTS

1. Frequent exposure to crowded situations—theaters, meetings, parties, department stores, and so on during winter.
2. Poor sleeping habits during winter. At least seven or eight hours required for most people.
3. Trying to do too much. Moonlighting and other fatigue factors are crucial to your resistance to flu during winter.
4. Lack of fresh air during the night. This is a must even in the dead of winter. Any window can be opened a little—preferably so as not to cause a direct draft on your bed.

WHAT MARK LEARNED ABOUT TOO MANY COLD REMEDIES

A patient I'll call Mark N. is a good example of what happens when you take too much of any of the so-called "cold medicines" that fill the TV ads today. Mark worked on a farm, and it was the corn picking season in September of the year. He had a cold with plugged up sinuses and a congested chest, and he was taking one cold capsule after another.

One afternoon, he inadvertently stuck his hand in a corn picker and lost all but his thumb and a little finger. In talking to Mark later, I found out he'd taken a double dose of the cold capsules, and the antihistamines contained in most of them had made him quite drowsy. He'd actually fallen asleep while standing next to the picker, and this caused his accident.

The moral to this case is to be cautious with these medicines. They do cause drowsiness and this can lead you to trouble.

HOW TO TAKE CARE OF SKIN INFECTIONS

Of all the infections I've seen in my lifetime, those starting from neglected, usually minor wounds of the skin are the most notorious for causing trouble.

This means that scrupulous care of wounds—all wounds, whether mere scratches or open and gaping wounds—can keep you out of deep trouble later on.

How to Treat Scrape Injuries

Wounds resulting from scraping on the ground are the most frequently neglected type of wound. You might get such a wound from falling from any object or just tripping and falling to the ground, where some of your skin is scraped on gravel, dirt or pavement.

Horseback riders, bike riders, skaters, and factory workers are most apt to get a scrape wound, though most of us have had one at one time or another.

Here is what to do when you get one:

1. As soon as possible after the injury, the area must be *scrubbed with a stiff brush with soap and warm water*. This should be done over the protesting you have or may hear from the injured party, and should be done until all the ground-in dirt and foreign matter is removed. This may take some real scrubbing, but do it. You'll be sorry if you don't.

2. Then thoroughly flood the area liberally with fresh hydrogen peroxide. (If peroxide has gone flat—that is, it doesn't bubble and fizz on contact with the wound—it's no good and should be replaced).

3. Cover the area with a loose bandaid or any dressing to protect from re-injury for a few days.

Jan's Bicycle Accident

The last patient I saw who failed to follow the above routine after a scrape on her elbow from having fallen from a bicycle, deeply regretted not having done so. Her name is Jan P. and she presented herself to my office about five days after the injury. Jan had blood poisoning in her arm that involved the tissues from her elbow to her shoulder. She had a temperature of 102 degrees and was almost delirious. Only hospitalization, antibiotics, and continuous hot packs, and her own strong constitution saved Jan. And all because the wound was "too sore" to scrub up after she had done it!

How to Treat Scratch Injuries

The same routine applies here, even to a small scratch, as applies above to the scrape injury, except a brush is rarely required. If you see redness developing around a neglected scratch, pus coming out of the bottom of the scratch, or red streaks running from the scratch toward your upper body, you'll know you didn't clean well enough!

The Treatment of Gaping Wounds

Any wound that makes the edges of the skin part, exposing the yellow "cobblestone" fat beneath the skin, or the red "meaty" muscle means that the wound must be closed so it will heal properly.

If you have such a wound and you find yourself removed from medical help for any appreciable time, here is a good way to deal with it temporarily.

1. Wash thoroughly with soap and water. Best method here is not to scrub—as in scratches or scrapes—but to flood the wound by pouring soap and water directly into the wound and letting the current carry it in and out, together with the dirt and germs, hopefully.

2. You can safely irrigate—or flood—the wound with peroxide as well. This will sting and burn, but can be tolerated. It will help clean out the wound.

3. Then take some thin strips of ordinary adhesive tape about an inch or two long. Dry the skin around the wound thoroughly. Fix one end of one of the strips on one side of the wound, and pull the remainder of the adhesive strip over and across the wound and fix it to the other side when you see that the wound edges have come together. Sometimes one strip will be enough; sometimes three or four will be required, depending on the length of the wound.

4. You can then cover the wound with clean gauze and keep pressure on it with plastic tape until you can reach a doctor. If you've done a good job, the doctor may not have to do anything else.

How to Avoid Lockjaw

In general, what about tetanus shots? These are the shots that you're supposed to have had as a child as part of your routine immunization program. They protect against lockjaw. What if you've not had them? The answer is that you should have them done now, especially if you work in a situation where dirty wounds are a common occurrence.

The routine is painless and takes a series of three injections spaced about six weeks apart. If you've already had this initial series of three tetanus shots in the past, a simple booster (one shot) will protect you against this disease (commonly called lockjaw).

When should you receive a booster? After any deep or penetrating dirty wound. Minor scratches, scrapes and etc., especially when they can be thoroughly cleaned out, do not require a booster for tetanus.

A booster for tetanus lasts up to ten years. Only major wounds that are especially dirty require a booster for tetanus sooner.

How to Manage Bleeding

Wounds that bleed usually can be controlled well by simply applying firm pressure *directly over the wound*. This can be done with your fingers or hand with a clean towel or gauze between the wound and your fingers. I've yet to see any wound, including those where arteries have been cut, that can't be controlled satisfactorily with this direct wound pressure. I suppose there are times when tourniquets are required. Short of the battle field, however, my experience has proved them unnecessary.

Serious Wounds

The one thing to recall with serious wounds—wounds that involve abdominal or chest penetration—is that all you need to do is to cover them thoroughly and snugly with lots of gauze or a towel and plenty of adhesive. This will do until medical help is reached.

HOW TO DEAL WITH BLOOD VESSEL INFECTIONS

The best treatment for blood vessel infections, commonly called phlebitis, lymphangitis (blood poisoning) or thrombosis, lies in preventing them in the first place.

Once phlebitis or lymphangitis has started, here's what to do:

1. The limb involved (and 99% of such infections occur in the leg or arm) should be elevated on a stool or another chair when you sit down. Don't let it hang or be crossed.

2. On four occasions a day, hot moist towels should be wrapped around the limb starting at the beginning of the red streak (involved vein) or below it, and extending up the leg or arm to at least eight or ten inches above the red streak. As the hand towels (the best for wrapping) begin to cool off, they should be replaced by warm ones simmering in a pan or skillet on the stove. This should be kept up for 30 minutes.

3. Following and between hot packing, the limb should be wrapped with a cotton or an "Ace" elastic type bandage. This is a rolled dressing usually of some kind of stretch material. In wrapping a leg, start where the toes join your foot and come up the leg to well above the trouble area (just as previously described with varicose veins). The wrap should be snug but not so tight as to cut off circulation.

4. When on your feet, *keep moving. Do not stand around on your feet!*

5. Some people still like to put patients with thrombophlebitis (inflammation of veins) on anticoagulant medicines. In my opinion, most of them do just as well without these drugs.

6. If your leg or arm is quite tender, and the bedclothes irritate at night, make a "cradle" of stiff cardboard that stands on the bed beneath the bedclothes, but over your arm or leg. This way, nothing will touch the involved limb.

If the vein irritation started with an infected sore or wound, your medical adviser may also want to put you on antibiotics for a time to further aid the healing.

Remember: There is no danger from blood clots breaking off inside irritated, inflamed veins if they are close enough to the surface of your skin to be seen. The dangerous ones are the *deep* veins. These can form clots. Often deep veins give no warning that they are inflamed and the clot will occur before you have time to treat the area. This is why I earlier stressed *prevention.*

A LIST OF THINGS THAT BRING ON DEEP VEIN TROUBLES

1. Prolonged inactivity from any cause. Long periods of driving a car; prolonged bed rest from any illness.

2. Taking certain drugs (recall what I said earlier about the pill for birth control).

3. Being too fat and not in good physical condition (read Chapters 2 and 3 again).

HOW TO DEAL WITH STREP INFECTIONS

The most common site of strep infection is in the throat—in the tonsils or on the sides and back wall of your throat. Strep can also cause infections in the middle ear, in dirty wounds, in sinuses, in kidneys, and in the blood stream.

When Your Throat Is Involved

Symptoms: Usually abrupt onset. Fever (101-103 degrees) with chills. Very sore throat, especially when swallowing; painful lymph nodes (felt as sore lumps) beneath the angle of the jaws and down the sides of the neck. General weakness and headache are frequent. Often pink or red flush in both cheeks.

Treatment: An excellent situation for penicillin. If you're allergic to penicillin your medical adviser may select another antibiotic to which you don't react. Rest in bed for at least 24 to 36 hours with isolation from other people as much as you can. No strenuous physical activity for a week. Warm saline gargles—dissolve one to three teaspoonsful of salt in a third of a glass of warm water and gargle frequently. Can also use peroxide as a gargle with or without salt.

Aspirin—two tablets every two or three hours as necessary. Warm packs to neck if lymph nodes are large and sore. (Same technique as with thrombosis already described).

When Your Ear Is Involved

Middle ear infections are commonly caused by strep, though not always. Ear infections usually start with a severe pain in the ear involved (usually only one side is involved at one time) that seems to be inside or deep in the ear. It can follow a cold or strep throat because the tube that drains the middle ear into the throat may have been blocked, trapping the germs inside the tube.

Pain builds up to an intolerable level rapidly. This is time for medical advice, for if not obtained at this time, your eardrum may perforate (draining ear) with possible future damage to hearing on this side.

A patient I know named Joan Y. comes to mind as someone in whom repeated infections in her right ear came along, with repeated bouts of strep throat in very enlarged, pussy tonsils. She refused to have her tonsils removed, thereby removing the source of strep infections. In about a year, Joan's draining right ear failed to heal properly. She went stone deaf on this side. She had to have extensive plastic reconstruction of her eardrum, but has never had quite the same hearing as before.

Moral: If possible, have the source of such strep infections removed surgically.

When Your Kidney Is Involved

Strep infections in the kidney aren't rare. They, too, usually follow on the heels of a strep throat or ear. But they can arise by themselves.

Symptoms: One sided flank pain, with pain radiating to the front of your abdomen across one side and sometimes down to the pubic bone. If you ask someone to jar the area at a point where your lower ribs join your backbone, exquisite tenderness at this point (either right or left) almost certainly indicates an infection in your kidney. You may also be spiking a fever and feel rotten in general.

Treatment: Again, a bona fide situation for an antibiotic. It will take longer for a cure here, so you may have to spend two to three times as long on the medicine as with a strep throat or ear.

The forcing of fluids is essential. As much liquid as can be comfortably pushed down during the day (every 30 minutes) to start that flushing action already described in an earlier chapter.

HOW TO TELL WHEN DRUG THERAPY IS NECESSARY

When is drug therapy needed? How do you tell? These questions are asked frequently and are very good questions. A few rules of thumb will aid you in deciding when, and under what circumstances antibiotic therapy is needed:

1. Most eye infections do better on antibiotic therapy. Most doctors use drops and/or special eye ointments containing antibiotics. Your eyes are quite indispensable and therefore, it pays to "go all the way" with any trouble that may develop with them.

2. Few sinus infections require antibiotics. The signs that may occur that foretell trouble and in which your medical adviser may use antibiotics are:

a. The appearance of green or thick, deep yellow drainage from the sinus cavities via the nose after previously having been clear and thin.

b. The spiking of significant fever to 101-102 degrees after sinuses have been acting up for awhile.

c. Exquisitely tender bony surfaces overlying any of the sinus cavities. You can tell this by pressing over your cheekbones or over your eyes.

3. The only common throat infections requiring antibiotics are bona fide strep infections and the more unusual staph infection. In both cases, spiking fever; enlarged lymph glands in the neck; and a typical appearance of the throat tell the story.

4. All ear infections should be treated with antibiotics. Hopefully at an early stage *before* perforation of the eardrum occurs (the draining ear).

5. About one third of chest infections will need antibiotics. The decision here rests a lot on what your medical adviser knows about your previous health.

6. Most abdominal infections (rare except for appendicitis) will require both surgery (for drainage) and antibiotics for adequate treatment.

7. Most skin infections will not require antibiotics if properly cared for at the time they occur (discussed earlier in this chapter). The appearance of pus in the wound, red streaks running toward the upper part of the body, and enlarged lymph nodes near the wound sites are tip-offs that antibiotics may be needed.

Do I Sound Anti-Drug?

You might think in reading sections of the book that I'm anti-drug. I'm really not. What I do plead for and fight about with a lot of people is the *needless* use of any drugs (including antibiotics)—not the *adequate* use of them when they are indicated. There are few infections, for example, when antibiotics are required that do well on less than six or seven days of antibiotic treatment. Anything short of this is inadequate. Many infections require ten days to three weeks to be adequate.

POLLY'S EXPERIENCE WITH DRUGS

An example of this was seen in a patient I know named Polly Z. who stopped treatment for her strep throat after only three days. In a week it was right back and treatment started again. Again she stopped treatment on her own in three days. In two weeks she was reinfected again. The next course of therapy sensitized her to penicillin and she could never have the drug again under threat of dire consequences. Polly should have known better, but failed to heed the advice of her medical advisor.

WHAT HAPPENED TO QUENTIN

Yet another patient I know, named Quentin L., was being treated for an intestinal infection that involved a typhoid like germ. He too, failed to heed advice and stopped his antibiotics too soon. He ended up with the infection spreading to his gallbladder where it remains today—he's become a permanent carrier of the germ.

SUMMARY

1. Cold and flu can, to a large extent, be prevented by utilizing a few rules of common sense health. Once started, colds and flu are usually self limited and respond to conservative treatment.
2. Almost all skin and blood vessel infections are likewise preventable with the use of scrupulous rules of first aid *when the injury or wound first occurs.*
   After infections have started, further procedures may be carried out in your own home that will help cure them.
3. Bacterial (germ) infections each have their own peculiarities and methods of treatment. When in doubt in dealing with chills, fever, enlarged lymph nodes, or pus in wounds or on membranes, consult your medical advisor.

14

Helpful Tips in Treating
Diabetes, Thyroid Abnormalities,
Liver Ailments and Epilepsy

Sometimes diseases come along in spite of the best efforts to prevent them. A common medical affliction in this category is diabetes. In this section we'll examine the disease and you'll discover how to more effectively deal with this disorder of the pancreas gland.

Among other common disorders that aggravate the human body are thyroid problems, of which there are three or four common varieties. You'll profit by learning what these are, how to cope with them, and how to achieve health in spite of their presence.

Liver ailments also plague the organism from time to time. In this chapter you'll learn the common ones and how they are treated.

The disease epilepsy has still the stigma of "something not quite right in the head" attached to it. We'll set the record right on this disease and discuss its control.

HOW TO MAINTAIN BETTER HEALTH WITH DIABETES

The true incidence of diabetes in this country isn't known. It is known, however, that a lot more people (perhaps as many as eight or ten million) stand on the threshold of diabetes because of the way they've neglected their health.

What are all these people doing to head them along the road to diabetes? *Not keeping their weight in control!* If there is one predisposing factor to this disease besides heredity it's being overweight.

Classification

Diabetes occurs in three main categories: Juvenile, adult and late-onset.

Juvenile: May begin any time after seven or eight years of age up to late teens. Is usually rather sudden in onset and may be quite "brittle"—that is, it may vary in intensity from time to time and be very hard to control. This is because of the day to day fluctuation in metabolic demands in the body while it's growing.

Adult: The most common type. Occurs any time before age 65 or 70. May be slow in getting started (may be present for a long time before symptoms show up) or may be suddenly precipitated by any stressful event such as during some type of illness like influenza or pneumonia.

Late Onset: Occurs in people past their sixth decade. Is usually mild in nature and not difficult to control. Often discovered by accident.

Treatment

Diabetes is treated by two main routes: medicine and diet. Regardless of what medicine is selected in your case, you still need to be concerned about *getting your weight down to ideal!* There are occasionally people who lose weight early in diabetes. They are thin, emaciated, and they look chronically ill. These people are few and far between. *Most diabetes occurs in overweight people.*

How to Handle a Diabetic Diet

It's no longer necessary to laboriously weigh each morsel of food you eat if you have diabetes. This used to be necessary, but it is not any longer. It *is* necessary that you stick with some diet gauged strictly to your needs—to the energy you burn up on a given day at work; at home; on vacation. If you are a person who needs to lose weight, your diet will consist of *less* calories (energy) than you actually need during the day so that your body will burn up your stored fat deposits as energy for its needs. When ideal weight for you is reached on this diet, it may be made richer in energy.

If you are underweight, your diet will consist of *more* energy than you ordinarily need during the day so that your body will store this excess and manufacture more protein to increase muscle mass in your body.

When your weight has reached ideal levels, your diet is stabilized—that is, arranged such that it contains just about the amount of energy you need during the day for what you are doing.

How to Tell When Diet and Medicines Need Changing

Obviously, your situation will change from time to time. Any time, for example, that you run a fever from whatever cause, your body burns more energy. Under such circumstances you will need more energy (calories) in your diet and more insulin or oral medicine (depending on which you use) to utilize it. When the disease that causes the fever runs it course, you can go back on the previous diet and insulin (or oral medicine).

If you change jobs or go on a vacation where your physical activity is increased, you will need more energy and more insulin. If such a change is permanent, the changes in diet and insulin will be permanent as well. If only temporary, the changes will be in effect until you resume your normal activity or job again. Then the previous diet and medicine will hold you.

Another situation that changes requirements and energy and insulin is a surgical procedure. Your medical adviser will normally adjust things to account for this stressful period. Then you will return again to the normal diet and medicines when the stress of surgery is over. The same applies to most other situations that put undue physical or emotional stress on your organism. Examples of this might be a death in the family; loss of a job; trouble with the kids; and so on. These situations are usually shortlived but may require temporary changes on your part.

How You Can Adjust to Changes

How to adjust? This is why your medical adviser will keep telling you to test your urine on occasion even though you may be in good control most of the time. This testing of urine from time to time will alert you when changes are indicated. For example, if your urine consistently runs 1+ on the test tape that you dip in your urine specimen, then suddenly starts running 3+ or 4+, you need more insulin (or oral medicine) to compensate for the change. This change will be in effect until whatever it was that caused the change is no longer in the picture. Then you can *slowly* revert back to normal diet and previous medicine levels.

How to Use Insulin

Most people today use three types of insulin: NPH, Lente, and regular. Any of the Lente types of insulin can be mixed in the same syringe if necessary. None of the other types should be mixed in the same syringe, but if two types are taken, they should be injected in *different* syringes and in different parts of your leg or whatever part of your body you are using to inject your insulin.

If you're on NPH (which is the same as Lente) you will find that its peak action is early in the afternoon if injected first thing in the morning. This means that your "heavy" meal should be at noon to deliver the most energy to your system at the time when the insulin action is at its strongest.

Regular insulin, on the other hand, has its peak action about two hours after it is injected. It's perfectly alright to have injections of both regular insulin (if you need an effect quickly) and NPH or Lente (for more delayed action) as long as you use different syringes to inject.

Additional doses of insulin can also be given in the evening, if your bedtime urines are running a bit high on the tape test at that time. A bedtime snack will "cover" such evening insulin additions.

Your Physical Tone in Diabetes

A fact that seems to go unappreciated, by and large, in the treatment of diabetes is the well known information that people who have diabetes always fare better in *direct proportion to their physical tone.*

This means your disease is milder and less hard in the long run on your organism and that you will require less insulin or oral medicines when you've reached good physical shape! The reason for this phenomenon isn't clear as yet, but it's thought that muscle cells are able to utilize energy more efficiently and store their own energy in immediately usable form more easily in direct proportion to their physical tone.

This means that whether you are a borderline diabetic or actually have the disease, *you'll maintain far more efficiency if you keep yourself in top physical shape.*

How to Recognize Increased Insulin Needs

Your insulin intake will need increasing under a variety of

circumstances. I've already discussed some of them. Boils are a common condition. A boil is an infection localized to your skin. The appearance of one will usually increase your insulin requirements. The same applies to most other infections. The more severe the infection, usually the more extra insulin will be required. If you are on NPH or Lente insulin, you can start this increase based on what the test tapes show on urine that is tested in the morning, noon, mid afternoon, evening and bedtime. You can increase by 2½ units at a time. Or if the sugars are strongly positive, 5 units of additional insulin can be added at a time until control is reached.

A good rule of thumb to use with insulin increases is that when you reach an increase in insulin where your urine sugars seem to reach zero or only 1+, drop back by 2½ units—that is, *decrease* the dose that controls well by 2½ units. This way, you'll have fewer insulin reactions (otherwise known as low blood sugar).

If you can't get the insulin dose well regulated in a few days, consult your medical adviser.

When Less Insulin Is Needed

As you drop your weight in getting your health under control, your insulin needs will gradually drop in proportion. As you build up your physical tone, insulin doses will also decrease.

This is a good reason to allow your urine sugars—or at least two of them during the day—to stay at 1+ positive. This way, as your requirement for insulin goes down, the 1+ reactions will disappear and the tests will all be clear of sugar. This means you're ready to decrease your insulin dosage.

The same also applies to stresses and infections that are clearing up. Your increased insulin doses will have to be slowly reduced as you return to normal.

Whether you are increasing or decreasing insulin or oral medicines, remember that *gradual change* is the rule of the day. Never make drastic or sudden large changes either way. Always be conservative whether going up or down with insulin dosage.

The Place for Oral Diabetic Medicines

A lot of controversy has recently arisen over the value of some of the so-called oral hypoglycemic agents—the oral diabetes medicines. I've followed this controversy and have reviewed the cases of many people I know on them. I think, and this is my personal opinion, that the controversy is a bit overdone. I think there is a definite place for the tablet or capsule form of diabetic medicine. I think one of the most ideal places for them is the late-onset type of diabetes I mentioned earlier—the kind that comes on after 60 or 65 years of age.

At this time, this milder form of diabetes can be well controlled in most cases with oral medicines. This doesn't mean *all* late-onset cases can be controlled this way. But most of them can.

I think also that the general state of health can be a bit better controlled at this later age when the oral medicines are used as opposed to starting insulin at this time. For example, I find weight comes off more easily when an older person is taking oral diabetic medicine than when on insulin. Physical tone—that is, increased efficiency of muscle—comes along somewhat easier when oral diabetic medicines are used as opposed to insulin.

In a young diabetic person, however, it appears as though insulin will turn out to be the method of choice. Certainly, there is practically never an indication for the use of oral diabetic medicines in the juvenile form of diabetes.

The big controversy over the oral medicines is whether they are able to prevent long term complications even though diabetes may be well controlled. In my experience there are certain long term complications that can't be prevented by any method of treatment. Some others seem to do better with insulin. After age 60, I think the point is academic.

HOW TO DEAL WITH THYROID PROBLEMS

The main disease conditions that occur in your thyroid are overactivity; underactivity; inflammation and growths that appear in it.

Your thyroid gland is a small, potent gland lying at the base of your neck, in front. It has two main lobes or parts, one on either side of your windpipe, connected by a narrow bridge of tissue that crosses over the middle of your windpipe.

The thyroid is the controller of your body's metabolism—that is, it controls the rate at which your cells burn up energy throughout your body. You might compare it to the thermostat on a furnace in this regard. If the thermostat is set too high, your cells burn up more energy than your body can comfortably produce for the "fire." When this happens, your thyroid is overactive.

When it doesn't efficiently burn the energy your body produces for its cells, the "fire" dies down to a flicker. Your thyroid is then underactive.

How to Detect Thyroid Overactivity

When this situation occurs, your body metabolism is greatly stepped up. Everything works overtime and burns out the available energy.

A patient I know, named Nancy A., had an overactive thyroid (hyperthyroidism). Nancy began to lose weight in spite of eating "like a horse." Her pulse and blood pressure both went up. She noticed she sweat a lot and coudn't seem to sit still. She became edgy, nervous and jittery. Usually, a close look at the spot at the front of the base of your neck just above your breast plate bone will reveal that your thyroid is swollen—enlarged so that it protrudes as a bump in your neck. Nancy noticed this as well. When I took Nancy's blood pressure, it was definitely elevated. She'd attributed the signs to a nervous breakdown. When she found out it wasn't that at all, she was greatly relieved.

I put Nancy on a drug that neutralized all the signs of her thyroid overactivity, and within a week's time, she felt well, had gained twelve pounds and was no longer nervous. This, of course, did not mean she was cured. The medicine only held the overactive thyroid in check. It was now up to us to decide what to do to slow down Nancy's thyroid permanently. There were three options: to continue giving her potent drugs for the rest of her life; to have almost all of her overactive thyroid gland removed surgically; or to use one of the newest tools in medicines—a dose of radioactive iodine to "knock out" some of her overactive thyroid cells. This method is a product of the nuclear era we're in and it is quite effective. It has the advantage of not requiring surgery yet it does the job intended. We used this method, and all Nancy had to do was come into the outpatient X-ray department of the hospital one day, lay down on a bed while the radiologist prepared the special drug and injected it into an arm vein. That's all there was to it. No more drugs. No surgery. Permanent cure of her condition.

How to Detect Thyroid Underactivity

A patient I recall named Marvin C. was 46 years old, lived in a small town, was always in good health, and was the holder of a responsible job with a railroad. Actually, neither Marvin nor his

family can remember just when Marvin began to slip into his
underactive thyroid condition (hypothyroidism). It began slowly,
almost imperceptibly. Marvin began to slow down—couldn't walk
very far without winding. Couldn't walk fast even for short
distances. He began to put on weight even though his appetite had
flagged the past few months. His wife noted that his legs and
ankles, his eyelids and face seemed puffy looking.

The next thing that happened with Marvin was that he went
completely out of his head at work one day. Told his boss to "go
to the devil" and stomped angrily out of the office for no good
reason at all.

When I saw Marvin (at his wife's request) he looked dull and out
of it and seemed slightly psychotic to me. His appearance was that
of the extreme underactivity of the thyroid—a condition known as
Myxedema.

After only three weeks on small doses of thyroid medicine (to
replace what his own gland wasn't producing) Marvin became his
old affable, easy-going self again, and all the signs of puffiness,
weight gain and so on disappeared. He will have to continue taking
his thyroid medicine all the time, but will be perfectly OK as long
as he does so.

How to Detect Inflammation (Thyroiditis)

Inflammation (thyroiditis) is an unusual condition, though not
rare. No one really knows what causes it but it can occur as a
result of an infection in the head or neck, or even a virus infection
in the body anywhere.

I last saw such a condition in a patient named Barbara M., a 27
year old woman who otherwise had been in good health. She'd
noticed some swelling and tenderness in the front of her neck, at
the base, following a bout with a flu-like virus. She was running a
slight fever (100 degrees) but otherwise did not feel ill. When I
examined her, there was no sign of abnormality aside from the
tender, slightly swollen thyroid. She had thyroiditis.

Barbara responded to this without any treatment at all in about
two weeks. There were no ill effects. About half of such cases will
show some overactivity of the thyroid gland while the inflammation is present. It promptly subsides when the inflammation stops,
which it generally does by itself and with no special therapy.

What to Do About Thyroid Growths

By far the most common growth involving the thyroid gland is a goitre. This is a small, medium, or large lump involving one or both sides of the gland. It's smooth and regular and causes no trouble except for its size. Occasionally the size reaches such proportions as to make breathing difficult from pressing on the windpipe. When this happens, it should be removed surgically. If breathing is normal, there is no reason to do anything with the goitre unless its appearance is embarrassing.

A man named Bob T., who was 53 and in good health came to me with a slightly different situation in his thyroid. He had a growth which he'd noticed for some time—maybe two years. It started small, then enlarged to a "raspberry" sized lump on the right portion of his thyroid. It had grown to this size only in the last two months, having been felt by Bob accidentally at first, about the size of a grapefruit seed.

Any lump or bump such as Bob's, that increases in size, that involves only a part of your thyroid, and that seems isolated in the middle of what otherwise is normal thyroid tissue deserves investigation immediately.

In Bob's case, his lump was a tumor. It was removed surgically, and apparently all of it was removed since it hasn't returned three years later.

The Proper Place of Thyroid Medicines

Of all medicines I can think of, thyroid extract is probably the most misused of any. It is given for almost any and every sign and symptom in the world. A common thing it is used for is any patient who is overweight. Except for cases like Marvin's which I've just discussed where it is definitely shown by proper laboratory and clinical examination that underactivity of the thyroid is present, thyroid extract is *not* indicated.

In this connection, I vividly recall the case of a lady named Carol Y., who presented herself in my office the first time complaining of extreme nervousness, agitation, bad dreams, loss of appetite, insomnia and weakness. She was 38 years old and had no medical problems in the past except that about a year ago, she told me, she'd gone to a doctor for a weight problem. He'd started her on some medicines which included taking two grains of thyroid a day.

Thinking that if two were good for losing a little weight, four grains would be good for losing a lot of weight, Carol had started taking four grains a day. A month later, seeing no results with her weight, she increased this to six grains a day—a dose rarely required, even in someone who has had his whole thyroid removed by surgery!

Small wonder Carol had all these symptoms. When the thyroid medicine was stopped, so did all her complaints. And when Carol mastered health principles, she reduced her excess weight without any drugs.

In order to prove what your medical adviser may suspect about your thyroid, there are laboratory tests that can be done on your blood serum to verify whether your thyroid needs to be treated—they will tell if it's under- or overactive. These tests, combined with the clinical signs, are reliable.

NEW BLOOD TESTS FOR THYROID TROUBLE

It used to be that the BMR (basal metabolic rate) was used almost exclusively to tell about thyroid activity. This was a test in which the patient was made to breathe a specific amount of oxygen through a tube and the amount carefully measured. From this, thyroid activity was calculated. This method is very inaccurate and was found to lead to conclusions that later proved quite erroneous. The newer blood tests are much simpler to perform, far less susceptible to error, and at least as economical to have done as the old BMR.

HOW TO COPE WITH LIVER AILMENTS

Liver ailments are not uncommon. Most of them can be avoided, much to most people's surprise, Inasmuch as your liver is a vital organ, its top efficiency must be guaranteed or your health will suffer.

The most common liver ailments are: hepatitis, cirrhosis, and reactions to drugs.

What to Expect from Hepatitis

This affliction (also called yellow jaundice) is caused by a very small virus. It gets into your bloodstream primarily via two avenues: by injection and by uncleanliness.

Jerry D., a young man I saw recently, had been taking drugs. Among the drugs he was taking was amphetamine—commonly known as speed. After the initial kick from taking this drug orally wears off, the drug user may resort, as Jerry did, to mixing a little of the powdered form of the drug in water or alcohol to dissolve it, then sucking the mixture up into a syringe and injecting it into a vein. This shooting of drugs is common among young people who are on the drug kick. Trouble is, they usually forget or just don't know about sterile technique—that is, making certain the needle they use is sterile and the syringe they use is the same. Hepatitis is a common result of such practice among drug users. Jerry came to me with yellow eyes, nausea and vomiting, weight loss, and extreme weakness. He had hepatitis from using dirty needles and syringes.

Other Hepatitis Transmission Causes

Dirty needles and syringes aren't the only way hepatitis can be contracted. In homes with poor sanitation, where washing hands after going to the bathroom to have a bowel movement isn't practiced, too well, hepatitis can occur. In any circumstance where sanitation in general is poor, hepatitis can occur.

Hepatitis, in fact, can occur even under the best conditions as with people who must have blood transfusions, for example. The donor of the blood may have had the hepatitis virus in his system and not have known about it. The virus gets into the blood he donates at the hospital and is transfused into the body of the patient accidentally.

This is why people at the blood donation centers are so cautious about asking whether you've ever had hepatitis. If you have, they won't take your blood. You might transfer the disease even though you've been over the disease for years.

This is also why people who must have injections—people with diabetes, for example, who take insulin—must always be alert and cautious about needles and syringes. Fortunately, today we have available sterilized syringes and needles in the bulk that are disposable—may be thrown away right after their use. This has cut down a lot on hepatitis.

The Key in Preventing Hepatitis

Still the disease is seen. It's seen where, as I've said, sanitation practices are not good. People using bathrooms that are dirty and soiled with feces are a common source of hepatitis. Crowded conditions where many people use the same bathroom, eating utensils, towels, and wash cloths are another situation inviting hepatitis.

The people who may be in intimate contact with a case of hepatitis, such as with the case of Jerry, should have the protection of gamma globulin—a substance derived from human blood serum that carries protection (antibodies) against hepatitis. But only the people in *intimate* contact need have these shots. The casual contacts need not fear hepatitis if they practice good sanitation.

Hepatitis seldom is serious, though it may be tough to throw off. Your system will do it, however, given plenty of rest, proper diet, and general supportive care. Jerry got over his case in about three weeks, and had gained back his lost weight in about six weeks.

How to Deal with Cirrhosis

Liver cirrhosis is caused in 99 percent of cases by too much alcohol. Alcoholics are therefore susceptible to cirrhosis. Especially alcoholics who have been heavy drinkers for ten years or more.

It's difficult to pinpoint the start of cirrhosis. It may simply be a feeling of something wrong after a good booze session one day—you don't get over the hangover like you once did. Then you may be aware of a fullness in the upper right side of your abdomen that persists. This means your liver is beginning to swell—it can't overcome the load of alcohol delivered to it to neutralize as well as it once could. You may notice lack of appetite; appearance of a slight yellow tinge to the whites of your eyes (as with hepatitis); the gradual change in the color of your stools from deep brown to lighter brown to almost white. And you may notice peculiar spots on your skin—especially around the face, shoulders and upper chest—that look like small, red, spider-like lesions.

How Chuck Stopped Progress of Cirrhosis

Chuck F. was a 50 year old man who'd been a heavy drinker for 25 years. He had noticed all of the above symptons when he came in to see me one day. Chuck and I had talked many times over the past five years about what his heavy drinking would eventually lead to. Chuck chose to ignore the warnings. He didn't even try to get help with his drinking, but kept right at it as though alcohol might soon go out of style. With the appearance of the signs of cirrhosis, Chuck at last became concerned. He stopped drinking completely, began to take good care of himself and got hold of his health through regular physical fitness toning, diet, and proper living habits.

Chuck was able to halt further cirrhosis (a kind of scarring in the liver, rendering it unable to perform its 20-odd functions), but was in his grave in five years from its effects. He'd just destroyed too much of his liver to maintain healthful longevity.

There is no way to reverse the effects of cirrhosis. There *is* a way to prevent it: Take alcohol in moderate amounts and maintain the principles of health we've talked about.

How Your Liver Reacts to Certain Drugs

The liver sometimes reacts violently to drugs you may take. The most notorious of such drugs are the ones being used by the millions these days: the drugs used to treat various kinds of mental illness.

This is yet another reason why I plead with people not to rely on potent drugs, if it can at all be avoided, to treat each and every sign and sympton they have. This is especially true of nervousness and the many symptoms produced by being unstrung and under too much pressure in what you may be doing.

HOW TO ENJOY HEALTH IN THE FACE OF EPILEPSY

That it is perfectly possible to lead a normal, productive and useful life with epilepsy is proved by a patient I know named Maxine L., who has had grand mal seizures (fits) since she was four years old. Maxine is the chief executive officer for a large bank in the town where I live. As long as she adheres to a few rules of thumb in dealing with what she realizes is a lifetime proposition with her epilepsy, she does quite well.

YOUR PROGRAM FOR BETTER CONTROL OF EPILEPSY

1. Be faithful in taking exactly the amount, every day of the year, of the medicines your medical adviser has you on to control your seizures.
2. Form a habit of drinking coffee. Caffeine seems to have an ameliorating effect on epilepsy.
3. Keep yourself normally hydrated, especially in hot weather, but don't overdrink fluids.
4. Women will notice a tendency to retain fluids near the start of their menstrual periods. Your medical adviser may put you on something for these two or three days of the month that will help eliminate excess fluids from your system so that seizures can better be controlled.
5. Go to any extreme to avoid situations that might produce a head injury. This is a good idea for anyone, of course, and may prevent you from having seizures (epilepsy often follows severe head injuries—sometimes a couple of years after the injury). Blows to the head are especially dangerous for people with epilepsy.
6. Epilepsy and alcohol don't mix. Except for a little wine now and then, your best bet with epilepsy is to avoid alcohol completely.
7. Activity, strenuous activity I mean, will not predispose you to more fits, but watch that you don't overdrink fluids with strenuous, sweaty exertion.
8. There are few epileptics that can't be controlled quite well with a proper combination of the drugs that are used for this purpose. If your seizures aren't well controlled on your present combination, seek expert advice so that they can be.
9. There is no reason why you shouldn't be able to indulge in all the tenets of health listed in this book just because you may have epilepsy. In fact, your disease will be the better off for having followed these health principles over the long haul.

SUMMARY

1. Diabetes in most cases is controlled well by general principles of health, in addition to insulin and/or oral medicines. More than anyone, a diabetic will reap benefits from a physical fitness routine in which all his muscles are toned.
2. Thyroid problems are fairly easy to spot and to treat, once recognized.

Thyroid extract medicine is overused in conditions where it isn't needed. Its only use is in the underactive thyroid.

3. You can avoid most common liver diseases by following principles of good sanitation and health, and by carefully preventing alcohol from getting control of your life.

4. Epilepsy needn't slow you down from practicing health control. In fact, your disease will be better controlled in the long run by maintaining your health in top performance and by being very careful that you use the proper anticonvulsive medicines your medical advisor prescribes, each and every day.

15

What You Can Do for Burns, Broken Bones, Shock, and Head Injuries

Among accidents that befall most of us at one time or another are burns and broken bones. In this chapter we'll talk about both of these accidents and show you what you can do with them, and when they require help from your medical advisor.

There are some special things that may help you if you must deal with shock and head injuries. You'll discover life saving aids.

HOW TO MANAGE BURNS

There is no such thing as a harmless burn. Burns, even though they may appear minor, are the most underrated of all injuries. The reason for this is that with any burn there is a loss of skin—and skin is vital to the maintenance of your body's health as I've already discussed earlier.

How to Handle Various Types of Burns

Burns are said to be first degree if there is only redness on the skin that has sustained a burn. This includes most sunburns, for example, though it's quite possible to have a deeper burn from the sun. The next deepest burn (the depth of skin involved is what determines the degree of a burn) is a second degree burn. Here, blisters form over the red skin. The blisters are filled with clear fluid (serum) from the deeper layers of skin. There are three levels of second degree burns, each a little deeper into the skin than the preceding one.

The worst type of burn is the third degree type in which all layers of skin are destroyed, leaving a charred, whitish, "dead" appearing defect where the burn occurred.

Managing First Degree Burns

This is the most common type—one we've all had from time to time, usually from overexposure to the sun, or from a hot stove, or from dozens of other sources. All burns are, of course, extremely painful. First degree burns are no exception. The skin "burns" long after the original insult and "fiery" red mark.

Preventing Sunburn

Ann G., a young lady I recall, overexposed her shoulders and back to the sun at the beginning of the summer. She wore a flimsy bathing suit and unhooked the chest straps of the suit to "get a more even tan." She neglected to use a sun screen preparation; she was a blonde and she underestimated the power of indirect sunlight since "the sun was under a cloud a lot of the time."

She was miserable when she appeared at my office from first degree sun burns on her shoulders and back. In addition, the whites of her eyes were quite bloodshot, indicating she had also burned them, as well.

The first thing I did was to cleanse Ann's skin thoroughly and gently with a cool solution of plain soap and water. The reason: *Any burn is highly susceptible to infection.* Then I covered a small area, mostly around her shoulders, with an anesthetic cream. This had the immediate effect of soothing down the most painful areas. Then I rubbed an antibiotic ointment into the remainder. This was to insure against infection. I asked Ann to wear an old, loose blouse without a brassiere. Her burn healed in about five days.

Abe Learned to Respect Steam

Abe L., a middle aged man, tangled with some steam from a heater he tended. His burn didn't fare so well. Abe received second degree burns on his arm and hand. By the time he'd arrived at my office, his upper right arm and hand were one solid blister.

I gave Abe some medicine to ease the pain, since pain is more severe with second degree burns. Then I cleansed the area—gently, so as not to break the blisters—with soap and water. Next I poked dozens of small holes into the blistered area using a sterile needle. You can sterilize a sewing needle for this purpose by holding it over a gas flame until it glows cherry red or by soaking the needle in rubbing alcohol. The needle punctures are made along the base of the blister near the normal skin. After the puncturing, I gently compressed the blisters—making certain I didn't tear them—to milk out the fluid. Then I put on a compression bandage to prevent the blisters from filling up again and to protect the very sensitive layer of skin immediately beneath the blister.

It is best to use Vaseline or an antibiotic ointment directly on the emptied blisters, then a layer of clean (preferably sterile) gauze, then apply the pressure with a roller gauze bandage or an elastic bandage or whatever is available to wrap it with. Safety pins will hold this outside layer securely.

The burn thus dressed can be seen for a dressing change again in about five days, at which time the blistered skin is usually separated from the exposed, bright red, deeper skin layers. This dead skin should be carefully removed with anything handy like tweezers dunked in alcohol (for sterility), and the exposed, deep layer of skin dressed exactly the same way as before. Gentleness is the watchword. I like to start antibiotics with most second degree burns that are more than superficial, since these deeper burns are notorious for getting infected. When they do, it makes an already difficult matter much worse.

Abe's burns took four weeks to heal completely, even without infection complicating the picture. This is what I mean by saying burns are the most underestimated wounds around. Always suspect infection and try to avoid it with scrupulous cleaning at the outset, and always expect two or three weeks healing time at minimum and be happy if it takes less than this. Many deep second degree burns won't heal even after six weeks of intensive care and scrupulous cleaning. These must have a so-called split-thickness skin graft applied to them for complete healing.

When Skin Grafts Are Necessary

This business of skin grafting isn't nearly so terrifying as it sounds and can often be done in the hospital outpatient department or even in the doctor's office if the proper equipment is available. A very thin piece of skin is removed from a "donor" site—say the thigh—and simply sewn onto the area of the unhealed burn. From then on it's treated like any other surgical wound and most skin grafts take quite well.

Virtually all third degree burns need skin grafting and this should be done in the hospital, where the burned patient needs to be under observation anyway. If you should have to take care of someone with third degree burns, just remember to cover them with a clean (sterile if available) dressing and treat the patient for shock (to be discussed in a minute) if there is any sign of it.

HOW YOU CAN ALLEVIATE SHOCK

I want to say something about this business of shock. In any accident or injury, it's apt to be present. If a person simply faints, this is the simplest form of shock. The most complex form of shock is when the patient remains unconscious, has a barely "takeable" pulse, and his breathing is shallow and rapid. In addition, shock makes the skin cool and clammy feeling.

The Treatment of Shock States

1. The injured should be on his back on a firm surface with his legs elevated. A chair or a stool will do for this, or a bunch of rolled up blankets or pillows or even a person squatting holding the patient's legs on his shoulders will do if nothing else is available.

2. Keep him warm. Even in hot weather, shock makes the body's temperature mechanism go haywire for awhile. The patient, if conscious, will be seen to be shaking as though from a chill. Combat this by wrapping with one, two or more blankets from feet to neck.

3. If the injured has a severe wound or is bleeding, the bleeding should be stopped if by nothing more than direct pressure on the wound with your hand and a towel or rag. If there is a bone sticking through the skin wound (as in a compound fracture), the leg or arm involved should be placed very gently, in a comfortable position, then splinted to keep the arm or leg from moving around.

4. Carefully watch his breathing if he's unconscious. If you see it stop, you can immediately begin to breathe for him by opening his lower jaw, extending his neck, holding his tongue down with a thumb or finger and exhaling your own breathe into his mouth (mouth to mouth resucitation) at about the same speed you ordinarily breathe.

HOW TO MANAGE BROKEN BONES

Whenever someone has fallen, twisted, bent, or otherwise wrenched a part of his body or when he has had a hard direct blow—like to his rib cage or head—you may have to deal with a broken bone.

Remember that it's never out of line to manage *any* injury as though there may be a fracture, until a medical adviser can take steps to find out definitely. You haven't done the injured party any harm by this, and you may save him a lot of grief.

How You Can Help Deal with Fractures of Arms and Legs

These usually happen with a fall to the ground or in an auto accident. When a child falls, the stress from landing on outstretched hands is usually transmitted up his wrists and arms into his shoulder where his collarbone gets fractured. This is the bone connecting the breastbone and shoulder. There is one on either side.

Inspection of a fractured collarbone usually shows a tender lump along its usually narrow and smooth course. This lump means the collarbone has been broken. All you need to do with this is to put the arm on the side of the broken collarbone in a sling suspended from the neck, so that the arm is bent at the elbow at right angles, and rests in the bottom of the sling without any pull at the shoulder. This relieves the pain and often serves as the treatment since collarbones heal without any special manipulation, as a rule.

I recall a youngster, a farmer's daughter, named Bonny N. When Bonnie was 14 years old, she had such a broken bone *about two months* before her worried mother brought her to see me because of the persistence of the bump at the broken site after it was supposed to have healed. I reassured her that all was well. At the end of a year, mother nature had dissolved the bump so that it couldn't be seen at all. Such bumps along collarbones that have been broken should be allowed to remain untouched for at least two or even three years. Most will disappear. Those that don't can be "chiseled" away if unsightly.

In an older person, a fall to the ground with outstretched arms might end with a severe pain in the upper part of his arm bone (about two to four inches below his shoulder joint). His arm is quite painful, almost impossible to move, and not much can be seen in the way of injury. When this happens suspect a broken bone in the upper arm (humerus). Sometimes such fractures can be treated simply by placing a heavy plaster cast from the middle of the upper arm down to the wrist and letting it rest in a sling. At other times, it may require more special care. At any rate, the use of a sling (snug and pulled well up to take the pressure off the shoulder) will suffice until your medical adviser can be consulted.

When the forearm bones (two of them) break there is usually a visible swelling at the break site because the bones are fairly close to the surface. As with most breaks, a bruising effect develops above and around this bump or angulation of the broken bones. This bruising on the skin is almost a certain sign that bones have been broken regardless of the area involved. A sling is good therapy again until help is at hand.

The wrist can be very tricky—after a fall, any persistent pain in the wrist should be investigated with an X ray. There are eight wrist bones and any one of them or the ends of either of the two forearm bones can break without much to show for it at times. If not cared for properly, a break in this area can result in a very stiff, painful wrist, so let expert help guide you in wrist injuries.

Hand and finger bones are usually swollen and deformed when they get broken. Finger breaks are also tricky. Some of them are easy to heal and cause no trouble later; others require a special reduction of the broken parts and proper splinting.

Dangers in Apparent Minor Injuries

I once watched an elderly lady named Dolores P. walk into the office under her own steam after having fallen at home three days before. Dolores was 72 years old. She couldn't understand why all the fuss was being made because all she had was, as she put it, a "little soreness around my hip."

Even on the examining table, not much pain was forthcoming as I moved her leg all around. Something told me I should X-ray this lady's hip anyway. I was glad I did. She had a complete fracture of the upper leg bone close to the hip joint. This shows how people vary in their response to pain and injury. Most people would have been unable to walk with such a fracture!

Breaks involving the upper leg bone and the two lower leg bones are likewise often difficult to see from the external surface, especially the upper leg bone. The leg bones are a long time in healing when broken, often taking twice as long or more, than smaller arm bones, for example.

Injuries of the ankle and foot can be tricky because they are surrounded by so many tendons and ligaments. It is quite possible to so severely sprain (tear) ligaments in your ankle that at first it could be taken for a broken bone. Such severe sprains should be under the supervision of your medical adviser because if they heal improperly, they can leave an ankle unstable, and then it must be repaired surgically.

Toe bones are probably the least innocuous of all broken bones, though they may also be quite painful. It is sufficient in most cases to simply wear a type of shoe that is comfortable to get around in, putting most of your weight on your heel when walking if necessary. Toe bones will heal well without fancy splints or plaster casts. If necessary, you can simply use crutches for a week or so until the pain subsides.

How You Can Aid the Patient with Knee Fractures

The knee joint is peculiarly vulnerable to injury, not so much from a break in the three bones that make up the joint (the thighbone and two lower leg bones) but because there is a situation in the joint where two large pieces of cartilage cushion the thigh from the lower leg bones. Given a shearing (twisting) stress to the knee, either one or both these cartilages can be torn, with great pain and disability later on.

Also there are two important internal ligaments holding the thighbone to the lower leg bones, and the outside of the knee joint is further stabilized by two sets of ligaments, one on the inner and one on the outer side of the joint. These ligaments are susceptible to strains and tears as well.

Therefore, by very cautious about dismissing knee joint injuries, even though they may not seem like much when they occur. Have your medical advisor check them out and follow them along.

Helping a Patient with a Pelvic Fracture

In auto accidents or falls, the bony pelvic girdle can be injured. These bones are so deeply covered over with thick muscles that they cannot be seen except at the very front where the two pubic bones come together at the pubic hair line and in the hip areas.

When pain with weight bearing persists and seems to involve the groin, the buttock, the inner side of the upper leg or the low back, suspect a crack in one of the pelvic bones.

Actually, unless the end of a broken pelvic bone has irritated or injured a pelvic organ (the bladder sometimes is prodded by such a break), pelvic fractures heal up with only rest which can be in bed or partly in bed, partly up and around as necessary.

Back Fractures

Broken backs are not all as dangerous as you might expect. They don't involve the sensitive spinal cord very much of the time, though when they do, it is one of the most serious kinds of breaks.

Usually, one of the projecting spines (what you can see and feel protruding down your spinal column) or one of the side "fins" of the back are involved. In falls where the individual lights on his tail from some distance, there may result a compression type break. This is where the body of one or more of the vertebraes gets squeezed like an accordian and has the effect of narrowing the body of the particular vertebra. These are not serious, and rarely ever cause injury to the spinal cord.

Most backs that are fractured are simply treated with bed rest.

Your Program to Help with Broken Bones

With any fractured bone, there are principles that will help you and the injured party until your medical advisor can be reached. Here is a list of these principles:

1. If the patient has to be moved, it is well to splint the injured part. By splint, I mean to immobilize the part that's injured so that the person can be moved without further damage.

With splinting, the idea is to keep things as simple as possible, as painless as possible, and to try to involve the joint above the injured bone and the joint next below it, if this can be done easily.

For example, if you have reason to suspect a hip fracture, the best thing to do is to lash together both legs with a pillow or two between them so that neither leg can move. Often, having done this, the patient can be carefully propped up for transportation without discomfort. He should be carried by two people to the car or ambulance, however.

If you want to splint a suspected broken bone in the forearm, for another example, putting the arm in a sling suspended from the neck with something to hold the folded arm in the sling snugly against the body will do. This also does for any injury from fingers to shoulder, if needed.

2. Over any swollen area (around a break), as long as the skin isn't broken, you can make things better by placing an ice pack while help is sought. This reduces swelling (therefore pain) and makes the application of plaster if a cast must be applied much less dangerous.

3. Medicine for pain may be indicated. You may have to use three or four aspirin. If you have anything with codeine in it, this will do an even better job.

4. If a wound is also present around a break in a bone (compound fracture), don't try manipulating the injured member, just cover it with anything clean (sterile, if available) to keep germs and dirt out. If such a wound can be immobilized as it is found, further damage may be prevented.

5. If the break or suspected break involves one leg, remember that just getting the patient on crutches may enable him to get to medical help without fancy splinting or other procedures. Anything that will get the weight off such a leg is indicated.

6. Recall what I've mentioned about shock. If the injured feels "fainty" or when he tries to move becomes nauseated and clammy (mild shock) keep him quiet until this wears off. If it doesn't wear off, transport him lying down rather than trying to make him walk.

7. Do not try using unwieldly pieces of stiff board or wood unless nothing else works for a splint. If solid pieces of metal or wood are used, be certain they aren't put on tightly—if you cut off circulation, you may do more harm than good. If there's any doubt, don't use stiff wood or metal for splints.

WHAT TO DO IN THE CASE OF SPECIAL FRACTURES

Involving the Rib

If a rib is broken, each breath may be painful. When this occurs, medical advice is generally necessary. I've tried the chest strap method in the past many times. This is where, with the air exhaled, the chest on the injured side is splinted by adhesive strips that extend beyond the midline in front and back (see description of this procedure in a preceding chapter). This is designed to keep this side of the chest from moving so much with respiration.

This is sometimes helpful, but proves bothersome as a rule. If pain is severe with a rib break it's better to let your medical advisor deaden the large nerve that runs along the underside of the injured rib with a local anesthetic. This is quick, stops pain completely, and requires no uncomfortable strapping.

In addition, if a rib is broken completely, the inside of the chest and its structures might get damaged. This requires expert medical care.

Involving the Jaw

If a lower jaw bone is broken, the only thing you need to do is to keep the jaw from moving until the dental surgeon is reached. To do this, simply tie a bandage made of any cloth from the top of the head around the jaw several times. Instruct the injured not to open his mouth to talk or eat.

HOW TO MANAGE HEAD INJURIES

Head injuries are a special type of injury because they can be complicated. There are some things that will help you in dealing with them. Here is a list of them:

When the Injured Person is Fully Conscious

1. Allow the injured to lay down until you're certain he's mentally clear and has nothing seriously wrong.

2. Care for any scalp wounds as any other wound. If any wound is gaping, it will do better if sutured closed. A simple dressing over it will suffice until help with the wound is obtained.

3. Observe carefully *any* head injury—from a simple blow without unconsciousness to a skull fracture with unconsciousness—for the following signs:

A. Any vision trouble. Black eyes.

B. Any bleeding from either ear. Any clear fluid oozing from nose or ear.

C. Any lapse into a stupor (sleepiness) other than at usual sleeping times. In other words, any loss of consciousness after previously being awake.

D. Any sign of one eye pupil being larger than the other—usually occurs on the same side of the head as the injury, if it occurs at all.

Immediate expert help is a must with any of these signs!

When There is Unconsciousness

1. Lay patient flat and treat for shock (see previous description in this chapter).

2. Make arrangement for transportation to medical help if unconsciousness persists.

3. If injured wakes up, same observations, only more critical, than with the conscious patient described above. If injured lapses into stupor again, waste no more time with observation. Get him to a hospital and expert help.

4. It is very unwise to try to get any liquids or food down someone who is not fully awake. Don't try it. Don't fool around with smelling salts either.

They aren't necessary and in a seriously injured, unconscious patient from head injury, will not work anyhow.

5. Observe breathing closely. If trouble develops, proceed as previously described under shock. Loosen ties, shirts, girdles, etc., to make injured comfortable.

Blows to the head and face often don't produce unconsciousness or serious injury. Frequently only a large "goose-egg" on the scalp is all that occurs. This means the small arteries and veins in the scalp are oozing. All you need do is apply ice to these bumps. They will disappear rather rapidly with ice packing.

Any wound that occurs inside the eye will require expert help. Don't try to fool with any such injury but get medical help. You may save such an injured person a lot of discomfort by simply patching the injured eye closed. To do this, place a small wad of cotton or other cloth over the closed eye and gently lay strips of tape or scotch tape across it from forehead to cheek. Instruct him to keep both eyes closed during this patching. When you're through applying the patch, ask him to open his uninjured eye—he should be able to see nothing through the patched side.

SUMMARY

1. Burns are notorious for becoming infected. The most important part of treating any burn is to cleanse the area well with soap and water.
2. A state of shock can set in with almost any injury, depending on the person who gets it. A few simple rules of thumb will control most cases of shock.
3. Broken bones can be helped before medical help arrives by following simple splinting rules. Wounds occurring with breaks in bones are compound fractures and will require help as rapidly as possible.
4. Special injuries to the face, head and neck can be managed by common sense and by careful observation of vital signs.
   In any circumstance where question exists, medical help should be sought.

16

Guides for Your Continuing Common Sense Health

IDEAL WEIGHT FOR HEIGHT TABLES

Men

Weight in pounds according to frame in indoor clothing. Height (with shoes on—one-inch heels).

Feet	Inches	Small Frame	Medium Frame	Large Frame
5	2	112-120	118-130	126-141
5	3	115-123	121-133	129-144
5	4	118-126	124-136	132-148
5	5	121-129	127-139	135-152
5	6	124-133	130-143	138-156
5	7	128-137	134-147	142-161
5	8	132-141	138-152	147-166
5	9	136-145	142-156	151-170
5	10	140-150	146-160	155-174
5	11	144-154	150-165	159-179
6	0	148-158	154-170	160-184
6	1	152-162	158-175	168-189
6	2	156-167	162-180	173-199
6	3	160-171	167-185	178-199
6	4	164-175	172-190	182-204

Women

Weight in pounds according to frame (in indoor clothing). Height (with shoes on—two-inch heels).

Feet	Inches	Small Frame	Medium Frame	Large Frame
4	10	92-98	96-107	104-119

Women (continued)

Feet	Inches	Small Frame	Medium Frame	Large Frame
4	11	94-101	98-110	106-122
5	0	96-104	101-113	109-125
5	1	99-107	104-116	112-128
5	2	102-110	107-119	115-131
5	3	105-113	110-122	118-134
5	4	108-116	113-126	121-138
5	5	111-119	116-130	125-142
5	6	114-123	123-135	129-146
5	7	118-127	124-139	133-150
5	8	122-131	128-143	137-154
5	9	126-135	132-147	141-158
5	10	130-140	136-151	145-163
5	11	134-144	140-155	149-168
6	0	138-148	144-159	153-173

For girls between 18 and 25, subtract one pound for each year under 25 from weights given in tables.

REDUCING DIETS

Strict

Breakfast: One slice of bread—toasted or plain.
One egg-poached or boiled.
One cup (8 ounces) skim milk.
One small orange or ½ cup (4 ounces) orange juice.

Lunch: Three soda crackers.
Two cold-cut slices or ½ cup cottage cheese.
Four ounces (½ cup) skim milk.
Two tablespoons raisins or one small apple.

Dinner: Any amount of uncooked asparagus, broccoli, brussels sprouts or tomatoes.
One serving of beets, carrots, peas, turnips or squash (one serving equals 4 ounces or ½ cup).
Two slices of any meat, or ½ cup (4 ounces) fish, or two tablespoons peanut butter on crackers.
Four ounces of skim milk.
Four ounces pineapple, or two of any dried fruit, or ½ small banana.

Less Strict

Breakfast: ½ cup (4 ounces) cooked cereal of any kind, or 6 ounces

(3/4 cup) of dry cereal with skim milk.

One egg—poached or boiled.

One cup skim milk.

½ cup any berries, or ½ cup any fruit juice.

One teaspoon margarine (one square).

Lunch: Two slices of bread, or ½ cup cooked noodles or spaghetti.

Two frankfurters, or two slices cheddar cheese.

½ cup skim milk.

Two cups any berries, or one peach or one apple, or two pieces of dried fruit.

One tablespoon cream, or one teaspoon mayonnaise.

Dinner: Any amount of uncooked cabbage, cauliflower, eggplant, greens or squash.

One serving of onions, turnips or carrots.

½ cup cooked rice, or two slices of bread, or one baked potato.

Three slices of any meat or cheese, or 3/4 cup of any fish.

½ cup skim milk.

¼ of any melon, or a dozen grapes, or two pieces of any dried fruit.

Two tablespoons salad dressing, or two teaspoons cooking fat, or two squares margarine.

At any meal or at any time between meals, the following foods may be taken in any quantity since they have negligible calories:

Coffee

Tea

Clear Broth

Bouillon (fat-free)

Dry Mustard

Any sugar substitute

Vinegar

Low Calorie Soft Drinks

Lemons

Unsweetened Gelatin

Rennet Tablets

Unsweetened Cranberries

Unsweetened Pickles

Spices

Seasonings

In addition, the following vegetables may be used at any meal or between meals so long as they are eaten uncooked:

Asparagus	Eggplant	Mustard	Romaine
Broccoli	Escarole	String Beans	Radishes
Brussels Sprouts	Greens	Spinach	Watercress
Cabbage	Parsley	Turnip Greens	Tomatoes
Poke	Chard	Lettuce	Rhubarb
Sauerkraut	Collards	Mushrooms	Peppers

Chicory	Dandelion	Okra	Celery
Cucumber	Kale	Summer Squash	

As you continue to diet, you'll learn how to substitute. For example, if you don't eat fruit for breakfast, you can substitute one strip of bacon from which the grease has been drained. If you don't eat bread or toast, crackers can be substituted. If you'd rather have all bread or toast, cereal can be eliminated. But no cheating! In general, meats should be baked, broiled, or boiled. Don't fry them in oil or fats. If you do use oil or fats for preparing meats, eliminate both bread and margarine from the allowable foods that meal.

When preparing vegetables from the cooked list, don't add flour or extra fat to them. It isn't necessary to use special foods. If you like canned fruit, buy it water-packed rather than packed in syrup.

Remember, it isn't wise to skip meals. Remember, too, that alcoholic drinks are heavy in carbohydrates—if you drink them while dieting, you must cut the amount of food at the next meal roughly in half to balance out.

Once you have your weight in hand, you may gradually slip away from your diet depending on your exercise routine. As long as your weight remains steady, you're getting enough to eat. If you have your weight steadied, begin your exercise routine, and find you're losing weight again, you need more food—don't hesitate to eat it!

The following is an example of a very simple reducing diet:

Breakfast: 1 egg.
2 pieces of bacon.
Fresh fruit.
½ slice whole-wheat toast and butter.
Coffee and cream or ½ teaspoon sugar.

Lunch: Fish or meat.
Green salad and 1.5 oz. vegetable oil.
½ slice whole-wheat bread and margarine.
Decaffeinated coffee or weak tea.

Dinner: Fish or meat.
Asparagus, or other low carbohydrate vegetables.
½ slice whole-wheat bread and margarine.
Green salad and 1.5 oz. vegetable oil.
Decaffeinated coffee.

STOMACH AND INTESTINE SOOTHING DIET

1. Strict Ulcer Diet (Progressive Ulcer Diet)

PROGRESSIVE ULCER DIET REGIME

Definition: A progressive diet schedule of smooth foods, bland in flavor, and containing a small amount of fiber.

General Instructions: This schedule progresses from hourly milk or cream feedings to a full bland diet for the convalescent patient.

Approximate Composition: See Suggested Meal Plan.

Bland #1. Provides hourly feedings of milk or cream.

Bland #2. Provides for the food allowed (see list) to be served at regular three meal hours plus nourishments. The meals on this regime are kept quite small. Unless specified by the physician, meals will be the same size as those on suggested meal plan. This diet does not meet the recommended daily dietary requirements for iron.

Bland #3. Provides for the food allowed (see list) at three regular meal hours plus nourishments. The meal size is somewhat larger on this regime than Bland #2; see suggested meal plan. This diet meets the recommended daily dietary requirements. (See suggested meal plan on following pages.)

Bland #4. If nourishments are desired in addition to this, they may be ordered by the doctor. This is a satisfactory diet for home use by the convalescent patient.

General Instructions:

1. Eat meals at regular intervals. Eat slowly and chew food thoroughly.
2. Eat three meals a day and add nourishment if needed between meals and before going to bed at night. It is much better to eat small frequent meals than to eat one or two large meals a day.
3. Do not chew gum.
4. Alcoholic and carbonated beverages are not included on this diet.

FOODS ALLOWED—PROGRESSIVE ULCER REGIME

	Bland #1	Bland #2	Bland #3
Beverages	Hourly as ordered—whole milk, skim milk, fortified skim milk,	Whole milk, buttermilk, cocoa, skim milk, fortified milk	Same as Bland #2.

	Bland #1	Bland #2	Bland #3
	cream or butter-milk.	beverages, chocolate milk, decaffeinated coffee, cereal drinks.	
Breads	NONE	White bread as toast, melba toast, rusk, white crackers.	White or light rye, melba toast, rusk, refined whole wheat, crackers—white or graham.
Cereals	NONE	Cooked: Malt-O-Meal, cream of wheat, farina, cream of rice, oatmeal, Petti-johns, cornmeal.	Cooked: same as Bland #2. Dry: re-fined such as corn flakes, rice krispies, puffed rice.
Cheese	NONE	Cottage, cream, American, Swiss.	Same as Bland #2.
Desserts	NONE	Plain, simple desserts such as: gelatin, custard, junket, corn-starch or tapi-oca pudding, angel or chiffon cake, plain cookies, plain ice cream, sher-bet.	Same as Bland #2.
Eggs	NONE	Poached, scram-bled, eggnog, omelet, souffle, creamed, soft cooked, baked, or shirred.	Same as Bland #2.
Fats	NONE	Butter or mar-garine.	Same as Bland #2.
Fruits	NONE	All juices and pureed fruits without seeds.	All juices, and canned or cooked: apples, pears,

	Bland #1	Bland #2	Bland #3
			peaches, apricots, cherries, stewed prunes, baked apples without skin, ripe bananas.
Meat, Fish, and Poultry	NONE	NONE	Meat once a day chosen from the following: broiled, boiled, baked, roasted or creamed chicken.
	NONE	NONE	Turkey, fish, liver, tender beef, or veal, or lamb.
Potato and Substitutes	NONE	White potatoes, boiled or baked without skin, whipped, creamed, steamed; rice, macaroni, noodles, spaghetti.	Same as Bland #2.
Seasonings	NONE	Salt, cinnamon.	Salt, cinnamon, allspice, mace, thyme, sage, paprika, caraway.
Soups	NONE	Strained cream soup of allowed vegetables.	Cream soups of allowed vegetables, chicken and turkey; strain all other cream soups.
Vegetables	NONE	Pureed only, may be served in cream soup.	Cooked tender green and wax beans, spinach, squash, beets, carrots, asparagus, peas, any other puree.
Miscellaneous	NONE	Small amounts of sugar, clear jelly, syrup, honey.	Same as Bland #2 Smooth peanut butter.

SUGGESTED MEAL PLAN–PROGRESSIVE ULCER REGIME

	Approx. CAL *2600** CHO *230* PRO *85*	CHO *230* Pro *100*
	Approx. PRO *63 gm* FAT *110* CAL *2300*	FAT *120* CAL *2500*
8:00 a.m. *Breakfast*	Administered by Nursing Department Milk or cream hourly 7:00 a.m. until 10:00 p.m.	Allowed fruit or juice Cooked cereal with cream Toast–butter Milk	Allowed fruit or juice Cereal with cream Egg Toast–butter, jelly Milk
10:00 a.m. *Nourishment*		Eggnog Toast–butter	Milk Crackers
Noon Meal		Egg or cheese entree–small serving Pureed vegetable or potato Toast–butter Milk	Egg, cheese, or meat entree Potato Vegetable Dessert Bread–butter Milk
2:00 p.m. *Nourishment*		Milk Gelatin Crackers	NONE
4:00 p.m. *Nourishment*		Custard Crackers	Custard or pudding Crackers
6:00 p.m.		Cream soup Pureed fruit or dessert Toast–butter Milk	Cream soup Meat Potato Vegetable Dessert Bread–butter Milk
8:00 p.m. *Nourishment*		Crackers with cheese Milk	Milk Crackers

SAMPLE MENU

Ulcer

Breakfast	*Dinner*	*Supper*
Orange Juice Scrambled Eggs	Poached Egg Buttered Canned Peas	Sliced Roast Turkey Buttered Rice

---

*Calories based on 2 qt. milk and cream (1/2-1/2).

Breakfast	*Dinner*	*Supper*
Cream of Wheat	Mashed Potatoes	Buttered Green Beans
Cream	Vanilla Ice Cream	Canned Peaches
White Toast	Milk	Milk
Butter	White Bread	White Bread
Jelly	Butter	Butter
Milk		

2. Liberal Ulcer Diet

LIBERAL ULCER DIET

Definition: This diet is modified in consistency by reducing indigestible carbohydrate and connective tissue, and in flavor by curtailing the use of strongly flavored foods. Also, coffee and tea are omitted, and spices and condiments are limited. It is served in three meals.

Approximate Composition: CHO, 225-250; PRO, 70-80; FAT, 100-120; CAL, 2300-2500.

The selection of foods include those mild in flavor. The lists should not be considered as restrictive inasmuch as food tolerance is a highly individual matter. Additions or subtractions should be made according to each individual's needs.

This diet meets the recommended daily dietary requirements.

Food Breakdown:

FOOD GROUP	FOODS ALLOWED	FOODS TO AVOID
Beverages	Milk, milk drinks, cocoa, Postum, fruit juices, lemonade, decaffeinated coffee; tea and coffee, if allowed by physician.	Alcoholic beverages, carbonated beverages.
Breads	White, light rye, finely milled whole-wheat, melba, rusk, white and graham crackers, biscuits, rolls, zweiback.	Cracked wheat, whole grain bread.
Cereals	Refined cooked cereals such as oatmeal, farina, Malt-O-Meal, cornmeal, grits, cream of rice, Pettijohns, dry cereals such as corn flakes, rice krispies, puffed rice, puffed wheat.	Bran and whole grain cereals.
Cheese	Cottage, cream or American	All others.

FOOD GROUP	FOODS ALLOWED	FOODS TO AVOID
	Cheese, Swiss cheese.	
Desserts	Simple, plain desserts, such as custard, gelatin, junket, cornstarch, and tapioca puddings, plain ice cream, plain cakes and cookies; allowed fruit, fruit whips, ices, cream puffs, eclairs, Boston cream pie.	Very rich or highly seasoned desserts. Desserts with nuts or coconut. Popcorn. All others.
Eggs	Any, except fried.	Fried eggs.
Fats	Butter, margarine, cream, vegetable shortening, mayonnaise, mild flavored salad dressing. French dressing, milk gravies, smooth peanut butter.	Nuts, coconut.
Fruits	Fruit juices; cooked fruits or canned: apples (no skins), apricots, pears, prunes, plums, cherries, pineapple, fruit cocktail, peaches, mandarin oranges; raisins in cooking; any pureed fruits. Raw fruits: (ripe and peeled) sectioned grapefruits, oranges, lemons, pears, peaches, apricots, avocados, nectarines, bananas, and plums.	All others; uncooked, dried fruits.
Meat, Fish, and Poultry	Steamed, broiled, boiled, baked, roasted, creamed, tender beef, veal, lamb, liver, sweet breads, fish, poultry, lean pork, bacon, glandular meats.	Fried foods; smoked, spiced, pickled meats and fish; luncheon or cold cuts, frankfurters, sausage.
Potato and Substitute	Baked, broiled, mashed, creamed or scalloped white or sweet potatoes; rice, noodles, macaroni, spaghetti, hominy.	Fried potatoes, potato chips.
Seasonings	Salt, cinnamon, allspice, mace, thyme, sage, paprika,	Pepper, horseradish, mustard, chili sauce, catsup,

FOOD GROUP	FOODS ALLOWED	FOODS TO AVOID
	caraway, vanilla extract, ginger, mint, parsley, almond extract, lemon juice, vinegar, nutmeg.	pickle relish, cloves.
Soups	Creamed soups made of allowed foods such as vegetable or chicken, oyster stew, homemade meat broths, consomme.	Any others.
Vegetables	Tender cooked asparagus, green or wax beans, beets, eggplant, mushrooms, pumpkin, carrots, celery, peas, spinach, hominy, pimiento, squash, tomatoes; others may be pureed or served in cream soups. Raw: lettuce, parsley, and peeled tomato if tolerated.	Any others.
Miscellaneous	Sugar, clear jelly, honey, syrups, plain candy, marmalade, and chocolate in moderate amounts.	Jam with seeds such as strawberries, boysenberries, raspberries, etc.

SUGGESTED MEAL PLAN

Breakfast

Fruit or Fruit Juice
Cereal with Cream
Bacon or Egg
Toast-butter, jelly
Cocoa or Decaffeinated Coffee

Dinner and Supper

Soup-crackers or juice
Meat or Meat Substitute
Potato
Vegetable
Fruit or Vegetable Salad with Dressing
Fruit or Dessert
Bread—butter
Milk and/or Decaffeinated Coffee

SAMPLE MENU

Liberal Bland

Breakfast	Dinner	Supper
Orange Juice	Roast Beef	Sliced Roasted Turkey

Breakfast	Dinner	Supper
Cream of Wheat	Mashed Potatoes	Butter Rice
Cream	Buttered Peas	Buttered Green Beans
Scrambled Egg	Soft Fruit Gelatin	Peeled Sliced Tomato
Toast	Vanilla Ice Cream	on Lettuce
Butter	Bread	Canned Peaches
Jelly	Butter	Plain Cookie
Milk	Milk	Bread
		Butter
		Milk

3. Colitis Diet

Food Group	Food Allowed	Foods to Avoid
Beverages	Coffee, tea, Sanka, carbonated beverages, cocoa, milk—one pint daily, including that in cooking.	Milk in excess of one pint a day.
Breads	Toasted white bread, melba toast, soda crackers.	Coarse grain breads, hot breads, whole-wheat bread, graham crackers.
Cereals	Cream of wheat, cream of rice, Malt-o-meal, corn flakes, rice crispies, puffed rice, most refined cooked or dry cereals.	Ralston, Roman Meal, Wheatena, Wheaties, All Bran, Bran Buds, all other whole grain cooked or dry cereals.
Cheese	American and Swiss cheese used in cooking only. Cottage cheese, cream cheese.	All strongly flavored cheeses.
Desserts	Plain puddings, ice cream, sherbets (these from milk allowance), gelatin, white, yellow and sponge cakes; sugar, vanilla and arrowroot cookies.	Pastries and desserts with nuts, coconut, raisins, seeds, and berries.
Eggs	All, except fried.	Fried.
Fats	Butter, margarine, cream, white sauce, mayonnaise, bacon, plain gravy or milk gravy from milk allowance.	Nuts, coconut.
Fruits	Canned or soft cooked fruit cocktail; peaches, pears, apples, peeled; apricots, bing cherries, royal Anne	All other fruits. No berries.

Food Group	Food Allowed	Foods to Avoid
	cherries, pineapple, fruit juices may be used. Baked apples without skins, ripe bananas, sectioned orange and grapefruit.	
Meat, Fish or Poultry	Tender ground beef, lamb, veal, poultry, glandular meats, lean roast pork, ham, fish. All to be roasted, broiled or baked.	Highly seasoned meats, such as frankfurters, salami, bologna, all pickled meat, cured and spiced meat. Clams, oysters and sausage.
Potato and Substitute	White potato, rice, macaroni, noodles, and spaghetti.	Fried potatoes, potato skins, potato chips, sweet potato.
Soups	Broth, strained cream soup made from milk allowance, vegetable soup if made with allowed vegetables.	Commercial vegetable soup, onions, and other highly seasoned soups.
Vegetables	Cooked asparagus tips, green or wax beans, beets, carrots, canned or pureed peas, pureed corn, chopped spinach, summer or mashed squash, tomato juice.	All raw vegetables, lettuce, celery, tomatoes, peppers, and onion.
Sweets	Moderate amounts of sugar, clear jellies, honey, syrup, marshmallows, hard candy, gumdrops, milk chocolate, plain creams, (if diarrhea is present, all sweets to be eliminated).	All others.
Miscellaneous	Salt, smooth peanut butter, paprika, parsley, vinegar, vanilla, cinnamon and mint.	Popcorn, pickles, spices, all seed containing jams, pepper, mustard, catsup, sesame, poppy, and caraway seed.

LOW FAT AND CHOLESTEROL DIET

Food Group	Foods Allowed	Foods to Avoid
Beverages	Coffee, tea, coffee substitutes, carbonated beverages, skim milk, buttermilk made from skim milk.	Whole milk, cream, chocolate flavored beverages.

Food Group	Food Allowed	Foods to Avoid
Breads	Enriched white, whole-wheat, rye, raisin, soda and graham crackers.	Breads made with eggs, fats and oils.
Cereals	Any with enriched or whole grain.	Cereals containing chocolate.
Cheese	Dry cottage cheese only.	All others.
Desserts	Cornstarch, bread, rice tapioca, junket, angel food cake, gelatin, sherbet, fruit ice, fruit whips, meringue, pastries, unsaturated fat pastries.	All others.
Eggs	Egg white only.	Egg yolk.
Fats	Corn oil, margarine, soybeans and soybean oil, safflower oil, peanut oil, vegetable fat based toppings and cream substitutes, salad dressings made with any foregoing unsaturated fats.	Butter, ordinary margarine, mayonnaise salad dressing, shortening, lard, suet.
Fruit	All fruits and fruit juices.	None.
Meat, Fish and Poultry	4-5 ounces meat/day: pork, ham, Canadian bacon, broiled, boiled or roast beef, lamb or veal, with no fat left on portions, chicken, turkey, most fish if packed in allowed oils (see above).	Bacon, brains, liver, sweet breads, heart, oysters, lobster, crab, shrimp, Fried meats, fish, or poultry unless fried in allowed fats (see above).
Seasonings	Salt, pepper, spices, herbs and extracts.	None.
Potato or Substitute	White potato, sweet potato yams, macaroni, noodles, spaghetti, rice, all with none but allowed oils.	None.
Soup	Meat broth without fat, bouillon, milk soups made with skim milk.	Cream soups made with whole milk.
Sweets	Sugar, jelly, jams, marma-	Candy made with cream,

Food Group	Food Allowed	Foods to Avoid
	lade, honey, syrup, molasses, hard candy, gelatin candies (gum drops, orange slices and marshmallows).	chocolate, or fat.
Vegetables	Frozen, canned or fresh.	None.
Miscellaneous	Chili sauce, catsup, pickles, vinegar, cocoa, olives, nuts, baking chocolate, non-hydrogenated peanut butter.	Gravy, milk chocolate, hydrogenated peanut butter.

If you are both dieting for weight and at the same time wish to be taking low cholesterol, the two diets can be made compatible by simply going through the above list and throwing out most of the fats and carbohydrates for your meals and substituting the allowable proteins until your weight is in line. Then, you may add some of the other allowable low cholesterol items to your diet.

DIABETIC DIETS

General Rules:

Measuring Food—Foods should be measured. You will need a standard 8 ounce measuring cup and a measuring teaspoon and tablespoon. All measurements are level. Most foods are measured after cooking.

Food Preparation—Meats should be baked, boiled, or broiled. Do not fry foods unless fat allowed in meal is used.

(Vegetables may be prepared with the family meals, but your portion should be removed before extra fat or flour is added.)

Special Foods—It is not necessary to buy special foods. Select your diet from the same foods purchased for the rest of the family—milk, vegetables, bread, meats, fats, and fruit (fresh or canned without sugar). "Special dietetic foods" should be thoroughly investigated and usually must be figured in the diet.

Foods to Avoid—Sugar, candy, honey, jam, jelly, marmalade, syrups, pie, cake, cookies, pastries, condensed milk, soft drinks, candy-coated gum; fried, scalloped, or creamed foods; beer, wine, or other alcoholic beverages.

Eat only those foods which are on the diet list. Eat only the amounts of foods on the diet. Do not skip meals. Do not eat between meals.

1200 CALORIES

Carbohydrate	125 gm.
Protein	60 gm.
Fat	50 gm.

DAILY FOOD ALLOWANCES

Breakfast

1 fruit exchange (List 3)
1 bread exchange (List 4)
1 meat exchange (List 5)
1 milk exchange (List 7)
Coffee or tea (any amount)

Lunch

2 meat exchanges (List 5)
1½ bread exchanges (List 4)
Vegetable(s) as desired (List 1)
1 fruit exchange (List 3)
1 milk (skimmed) exchange (List 7)
2 fat exchanges (List 6)
Coffee or tea (any amount)

Dinner

2 meat exchanges (List 5)
1½ bread exchanges (List 4)
Vegetables as desired (List 1)
1 vegetable exchange (List 2)
1 fruit exchange (List 3)
1 fat exchange (List 6)
Coffee or tea (any amount)

LIQUID DIETS
(May be used to replace any one of the meals)

Full Liquid

Eggnog—milk—½ cup	
egg—1	120 gm.
Orange Juice—1 cup	240 gm.
Milk—3/4 cup	150 gm.

Clear Liquid

Clear Bouillion—1 cup	
Orange Juice—1 cup	240 gm.
Grapefruit Juice—½ cup	120 gm.
Gelatin dessert—½ cup	100 gm.

Bedtime Feeding

(Only when directed by physician)

½ milk exchange (½ cup milk) will add approximately

½ bread exchange (2 crackers) 120 calories to daily diet.

FOODS ALLOWED AS DESIRED

List 1—Need Not Be Measured

Seasonings: Cinnamon, celery salt, garlic, garlic salt, lemon, mustard, mint, nutmeg, parsley, pepper, saccharin and other sugarless sweeteners, spices, vanilla, and vinegar.

Other Foods: Coffee or tea (without sugar or cream), fat-free broth, unflavored gelatin, rennet tablets, sour or dill pickles, cranberries (without sugar), rhubarb (without sugar).

Vegetables: Group A—insignificant carbohydrate or calories. You may eat as much as desired of raw vegetable. If cooked vegetable is eaten, limit amount to 1 cup.

Asparagus	Lettuce
Broccoli	Mushrooms
Brussels Sprouts	Okra
Cabbage	Peppers, green or red
Cauliflower	Radishes
Celery	Sauerkraut
Chicory	String Beans
Cucumber	Summer Squash
Eggplant	Tomatoes
Escarole	Watercress

Green: Beet, chard, collard, dandelion, kale, mustard, spinach, turnip.

Other foods allowed, see lists 2 through 7.

List 2—Vegetable Exchanges

Carbohydrate, 7 gm.

Protein, 2 gm.   Calories—36

Vegetables: Group B—One serving equals ½ cup, or 100 gm.

Beets	Pumpkin
Carrots	Rutabagas
Onions	Squash, winter
Peas, green	Turnips

List 3—Fruit Exchanges

(fresh or canned without sugar)

Carbohydrate, 10 gm.   Calories—40

Apple	1 small (2" diam.)	80 gm.
Applesauce	½ cup	100 gm.
Apricots, fresh	2 med.	100 gm.
Apricots, dried	4 halves	20 gm.
Banana	½ small	50 gm.
Berries	1 cup	150 gm.
Blueberries	2/3 cup	100 gm.
Cantaloupe	¼ (6") diam.)	200 gm.
Cherries	10 large	75 gm.
Dates	2	15 gm.
Figs, fresh	2 large	50 gm.
Figs, dried	1 small	15 gm.
Grapefruit	½ small	125 gm.
Grapefruit Juice	½ cup	100 gm.
Grapes	12	75 gm.
Grape Juice	¼ cup	60 gm.
Honeydew Melon	1/8 (7" diam.)	150 gm.
Mango	½ small	70 gm.
Orange	1 small	100 gm.
Orange Juice	½ cup	100 gm.
Papaya	1/3 medium	100 gm.
Peach	1 medium	100 gm.
Pear	1 small	100 gm.
Pineapple	½ cup	80 gm.
Pineapple Juice	1/3 cup	80 gm.
Plums	2 medium	100 gm.
Prunes, dried	2	25 gm.
Raisins	2 tbsp.	15 gm.
Tangerine	1 large	100 gm.
Watermelon	1 cup	175 gm.

List 4—Bread Exchanges

Carbohydrate, 15 gm.

Protein, 2 gm.   Calories—68

Bread	1 slice	25 gm.
Biscuit, roll	1 (2" diam.)	35 gm.
Muffin	1 (2" diam.)	35 gm.
Cornbread	1 ½" cube	35 gm.
Flour	2½ tbsp.	20 gm.
Cereal, cooked	½ cup	100 gm.
Cereal, dry (flakes or puffed)	3/4 cup	20 gm.
Rice or grits, cooked	½ cup	100 gm.
Spaghetti, noodles, etc.	½ cup	100 gm.
Crackers, graham	2	20 gm.

Crackers, Oyster	20 (½ cup)	20 gm.
Crackers, Saltine	5	20 gm.
Crackers, soda	3	20 gm.
Crackers, round	6-8	20 gm.
Vegetables		
Beans (Lima, navy, etc.) cooked	½ cup	90 gm.
Peas (split peas, etc.) dry, cooked	½ cup	90 gm.
Baked beans, no pork	¼ cup	50 gm.
Corn	1/3 cup	80 gm.
Parsnips	2/3 cup	125 gm.
Potatoes, white, baked or boiled	1 (2" diam.)	100 gm.
Potatoes; white, mashed	½ cup	100 gm.
Potatoes, sweet, or Yams	¼ cup	50 gm.
Sponge Cake, plain	1 ½" cube	25 gm.
Ice cream (omit 2 fat exchanges)	½ cup	70 gm.

List 5—Meat Exchanges

Protein, 7 gm.

Fat, 5 gm.   Calories—73

30 gm. equals 1 ounce

Meat and poultry (beef, lamb, pork, liver, chicken, etc.)

Medium Fat	1 slice (3" x 2" x 1/8")	30 gm.
Cold Cuts	1 slice (4½" sq. 1/8" thick)	45 gm.
Frankfurter	1 (8-9 per lb.)	50 gm.
Codfish, mackerel, etc.	1 slice (2" x 2" x 1")	30 gm.
Salmon, tuna, crab	¼ cup	30 gm.
Oysters, shrimp, clams	5 small	45 gm.
Sardines	3 medium	30 gm.
Cheese, cheddar, American	1 slice (3½" x 1½" x ¼")	30 gm.
Cheese, cottage	¼ cup	45 gm.
Egg	1	50 gm.
Peanut Butter	2 tbsp.	30 gm.

Limit peanut butter to one exchange per day unless carbohydrate is allowed for in diet plan.

List 6—Fat Exchanges

Fat, 5 gm.   Calories—45

Butter or margarine	1 tsp.	5 gm.
Bacon, crisp	1 slice	10 gm.
Cream, light	2 tbsp.	30 gm.
Cream, heavy	1 tbsp.	15 gm.
Cream cheese	1 tbsp.	15 gm.
French dressing	1 tbsp.	15 gm.
Mayonnaise	1 tsp.	5 gm.

Oil or cooking fat	1 tsp.	5 gm.
Nuts	6 small	10 gm.
Olives	5 small	50 gm.
Avocado	1/8 (4" diam.)	25 gm.

List 7—Milk Exchanges

Carbohydrate, 12 gm.
Protein, 8 gm.   Calories—170
Fat, 10 gm.

Milk, whole	1 cup	240 gm.
Milk, evaporated	½ cup	120 gm.
Milk, powdered	¼ cup	35 gm.
Buttermilk	1 cup	240 gm.

Add two fat exchanges if milk is fat-free.

Sample menus below illustrate use of Exchange Lists provided above.

MENU #1

Breakfast

Orange Juice	½ cup
Toast	1 slice
Egg	1
Milk, whole	1 cup

Lunch

Meat	2 slices (3" x 2" x 1/8" ea.)
Potatoes	½ cup
Lettuce and tomato salad	as desired
Bread	½ slice
Butter	1 tsp.
Pineapple	½ cup
Milk, skimmed	1 cup
French dressing	1 tbsp.

Dinner

Tomato Juice	3 oz.
Chicken	2 slices (3" x 2" x 1/8" ea.)
Noodles	½ cup
Asparagus	as desired
Peas	½ cup
Bread	½ slice
Butter	1 tsp.
Banana	½ small

MENU #2

Breakfast

Prunes	2 medium
Toast	1 slice
Egg	1
Butter	1 tsp.
Milk, skimmed	1 cup
Cream	1 oz.

Lunch

Meat or cheese	2 slices (3" x 2" x 1/8" ea.)
Bread	1 slice
Butter	1 tsp.
Mayonnaise	1 tsp.
Coleslaw with vinegar	as desired
Grapes	12
Milk, skimmed	1 cup
Graham cracker	1

Dinner

Broth, fat-free	as desired
Hamburger	2 patties (3" diam., ¼" thick)
Potatoes	½ cup
Green beans	as desired
Carrots, diced	½ cup
Bread	½ slice
Butter	1 tsp.
Grapefruit sections	½ cup

1800 CALORIES

Here is an example of how to use the exchange list for 1800 calories:

Carbohydrate	180 gm.	
Protein	80 gm.	Calories—1800
Fat	80 gm.	

DAILY FOOD ALLOWANCES

Breakfast

2 fruit exchanges (List 3)
2 bread exchanges (List 4)
2 meat exchanges (List 5)
1 milk exchange (List 7)
1 fat exchange (List 6)
Coffee or tea (any amount)

Lunch

2 meat exchanges (List 5)
2 bread exchanges (List 4)
Vegetables as desired (List 1)
1 vegetable exchange (List 2)
1 fruit exchange (List 3)
1 milk exchange (List 7)
1 fat exchange (List 6)
Coffee or tea (any amount)

Dinner

2 meat exchanges (List 5)
2 bread exchanges (List 4)
Vegetables as desired (List 1)
1 vegetable exchange (List 2)
1 fruit exchange (List 3)
1 milk exchange (List 7)
1 fat exchange (List 6)
Coffee or tea (any amount)

SPECIAL PROTEIN SNACK RECIPES

Peanut Snack Rounds

2 Jars (12 oz. each) smooth peanut butter
1-1/2 cups honey

2 cups dry milk granules
1 cup chopped peanuts
1 cup raisins.

Combine peanut butter and honey. Add dry milk granules, peanuts and raisins. Mix until well blended and mixture holds together well. Shape mixture into two rolls, each about 12 inches long. Wrap rolls in foil. Chill. Cut in ½ inch thick slices to serve. Makes about four pounds.

Granola with Fruits

5 cups uncooked oats
¼ cup firmly packed brown sugar
½ cup salted soybeans, finely chopped
1/3 cup vegetable oil

1/3 cup honey
½ cup raisins
½ cup chopped, dried apricots
½ cup chopped dates
½ cup chopped walnuts

Heat oats in an ungreased 13 x 9 inch baking pan in a preheated moderate oven (350°F) for 10 minutes. Combine oats, brown sugar and soybeans. Add oil and honey; mix until dry ingredients are well coated. Bake in ungreased 13 x 9 inch baking pan in preheated oven (350°F.) for 20 to 25 minutes, stirring often to brown evenly. Add raisins, apricots, dates and walnuts. Stir until crumbly. Store in a tightly covered container. Makes about 8 cups.

ALTERNATE EXERCISES FOR VARIOUS MUSCLE GROUPS

Face

Your forehead muscles are controlled by the same ones that elevate your eyebrows. Practice in front of a mirror elevating both eyebrows to their fullest height, then pull down into a deep "scowl" position. Repeat this maneuver several times. Later, practice elevating both brows, then lowering just your left brow, then just the right.

When you can control either side at will, your frontal muscles will be in good shape, and many of those wrinkles will be ironed out.

The muscles around your eyes are important because they are the "bags" beneath your eyes when they're out of condition. These muscles also get the dark circles in them and cause you to appear ill. Exercise these muscles by pulling up your cheeks toward your eyes and smiling broadly at the same time. With this forced "squint" held firmly in place, close both eyelids forcibly until you feel the muscles that encircle them pull tightly, then relax. Repeat this several dozen times.

The muscles that move your eyeballs around can be exercised by simply moving your eyes rapidly in all conceivable directions until your vision is blurred from the rapid movement.

The muscles that exercise your mouth are used simply by pulling your mouth into a forced smile and holding it for a few seconds. This can be alternated with an enforced droop of the mouth which also pulls your chin muscles inwardly. Alternately pursing your lips into a tight round puckered shape, then into lips turned outwardly, then lips pulled to the sides, will exercise the muscles that surround your mouth. Forcibly opening your mouth, utilizing the muscles beneath your chin, and holding this position will aid in getting rid of the double chin as well.

Cheek muscles can be toned by blowing both cheeks out while holding your mouth closed, then by sucking both cheeks inwardly so your lips are protruding out like a fish.

Neck

Neck muscles are often neglected in considering exercises. The three main groups of muscles to consider are the ones that turn your head right and left; the ones that bend your head forward to the chin-on-chest position and back to chin-turned-up position; and the ones that bend your head to the ear-on-shoulder positions.

The easiest way to exercise neck muscles is to position your head and neck in any of the six positions mentioned, then force your neck in the opposite direction against the resistance of your hand. For example, with your head turned to the left, turn it to the right against the resistance of your right hand lying alongside your right forehead. Bend your neck backward from the chin-on-chest position against the resistance of your hands clasped alongside the back of your head. Bend your neck from the left ear-on-shoulder position against the resistance of your right hand lying alongside your right temple. You can increase or decrease the pressure of the resisting hand. Since these muscles are seldom used, it's wise to take it easy at first—don't force too hard. Expect to hear some "creaking" of neck ligaments with these exercises—it's quite safe.

Shoulders

You can strengthen your shoulders in a number of ways. A simple isometric method is to elevate one shoulder against the resistance of the opposite hand pulling downward on it. Another way is to lean against a door frame with only your shoulder supporting your weight against it. Suddenly, make your shoulder forcefully push your body away from the frame. Reverse this by turning around and leaning against the frame with the back part of your shoulder and push away by suddenly forcing your shoulder backward.

Using a small weight is another good way to strengthen shoulders. Using a ten pound bell—the short bar that comes with weight sets with a five pound weight at either end—slowly elevate the weight from alongside your leg to a point where your arm is extended straight above your head, then back down again. Keep your arm straight at the elbow and make your shoulder muscles do all the lifting. Do this extending your arm forward, sidewise, and to the rear.

Another exercise for your shoulders is to use the long bar of the weight set with 20 to 25 pounds on either end. Place the bar on the floor with one weight in the direction you're facing, the other end to the rear. Now bend at your knees and waist until you can grab the middle of the bar. Keeping your legs and waist stiff, make your shoulder muscles pick up the weight until the bar is at the level of your chest, then return the weight to the floor. Repeat this as often as you can, increasing the number of times gradually.

If you have a punching bag, boxing the bag and increasing the time you hold your arms up to punch will give stamina to your shoulder muscles.

Chest

One of the bonuses of using weights is that when you grab a weight in almost any position, and lift it or change its position in any way, your shoulder, chest, arm and grip are all helped. The same applies to chinning yourself on one of the basement pipes. Whenever you pull yourself up to the pipe your arms, chest, and grip muscles are benefited.

Your chest muscles can be pulled by simply grasping hands in front of your chest, and pulling in opposite directions with your arms and hands. As you pull, bend your elbows inwardly toward your rib cage to tighten your chest muscles even more. There is nothing like swimming and tennis for chest muscle tone. Hand ball and chopping wood will also do nicely as variations in toning the chest muscles.

Arm

Alternate methods to exercise and tone your arm muscles will help keep the drudgery from your exercise routines. Try extending your arms against any flat wall, using your body as a counter-weight against them. Simply make your arms push you away (or pull you toward) the wall or door frame and press your hands against the top of the frame. Usually, you will find that your arms aren't completely extended. Now make your arms straighten out by pushing upward.

Any manipulations of weights while lying flat on the floor is an alternate to standing up and using them. Use the small weights and bar first. When you feel tone returning in your arms, you can switch to the long bar and more weights. Add weights *slowly,* and you'll avoid strain and unnecessary muscle knotting.

Rowing a boat is good arm and chest exercise. Sawing wood will also condition arm muscles quite well.

Abdomen

One variation to strengthen your abdomen when you've mastered the sit-up in the way I've described, is to do sit-ups with a small amount of weight in your hands. Use the small bar and light weights at first. Yet another variation is to do scissor kicks and sit-ups at the same time. This takes a bit of practice, but really keeps that abdomen in shape!

While standing, use a circular motion at your waist muscles—bend forward, to each side, and backwards, hands on hips and using a smooth motion. This keeps the waistline trim. With feet a bit apart, bend to one side as far as possible, arms outstretched, dipping the arm to the side toward which you bend. Do the same with the opposite side.

Suck in your abdomen until you feel yourself shaking with the exertion, then tighten down your abdominal muscles so that they bend you forward at the waist, hardening your abdominal wall so that you can forcefully dig both thumbs or fists into it without discomfort. This is an alternate isometric for your abdominal muscles.

Legs

Practice getting up from the floor and standing from a sitting position in a chair without using your arms to help. If you're on the floor, cross both legs, Indian style, then make them hoist you to a standing position without bracing with your arms. This tones up those thigh muscles. While standing, lean against a dresser or door frame with one hand, and reach behind you with the opposite hand to grasp your ankle, bending your knee so you can reach it. Now forcefully straighten your leg against the resistance of your grip on your ankle. This tones up your hamstring muscles—the ones that make the cords in back of your knee joint. Again, swimming, cycling and just plain walking does wonders for those legs. Enjoy the lift of spirit and feel the exhilaration of a brisk early morning or late evening walk.

FURTHER HELP TO EASE BACK PAIN

Bed

Bed rest is advisable. If you must work, try to arrange rest periods during the day. In any case, plan to spend more time in bed than you ordinarily would, retiring earlier, and resting on weekends. Use a firm mattress!

Board

A plywood board (3/4" to 1" thick) should be placed between the mattress and box spring. This will help lessen the strain on your back. If boards are not available at department stores, a local lumber yard can cut one to order.

Heat

Moist heat is preferred. Relax in a hot bath for 20 minutes in the morning and evening.

At other times, apply hot towels to your back. Repeat these applications two to four times daily.

SPECIAL FORMULAS FOR THE CARE OF YOUR SKIN
(To be filled at a Pharmacy)

Skin Problem	Formula to Use	
Recent Eczema:	Acetone	
	Flexible Collodion	aa 4.0
	Crude Coal Tar	QS 30.0 (Mix well)

Apply one to three times daily to affected skin.

Long Standing Eczema:	Icthyol	3.0
	Unguent	ZnO QS 100.00

Apply one to three times daily to affected skin.

Foot Skin Condition	Salicylic Acid	2.0
	Boric Acid	6.0
	Zinc Stearate	3.0
	Exsicated Alum	1.0
	Starch	10.0
	Talcum Powder	78.0

Use once to four times daily between toes; on feet; in shoes to keep skin dry.

Cold Sores (Canker	Menthol	0.25
sores or fever blisters)	Phenol	0.5
Outside of Mouth	Resorcin	3.0
	LCD (Liquor Carbonis Detergens)	7.0
	Zinc Oxide	20.0
	Glycerin	15.0
	95% Alcohol QS	60

Shake well and apply to sore. Let dry and remain in place. Repeat when necessary.

Scalp Dermatitis and	S.U.L.	3.0
Groin and Foot Fungus	Salicylic Acid	3.0
Infection. (Can often	Cetyl Tar Dist.	4.0
be found on shelf already	Duponol	1.0
prepared under name	Pertrolatum	38.0
Pragmatar)	Stearyl Alcohol	18.0
	Cetyl Alcohol	7.0
	Mineral Oil	25.0

Rub into affected skin once or twice daily following washing or shampoo and thorough drying.

"Weeping" Dermatitis (Moist-Oozing Types)	Aluminum Subacetate (comes in packets) (Also known as Burrow's Powder or Tablets)

Dissolve ½ to one package (or tablet) in 1 pint water. Make fresh daily. To use soak through gauze on affected skin once to three times a day until weeping stops.

Corns   Salicylic Acid
                 Alcohol $\overline{aa}$ 10-20%
                 Flexible Collodion QS

Paint thoroughly corn areas once or twice daily.

Barber's Itch   Quinolor Ointment
(Acute, irritated, itching
skin from razor nicks)

Rub thoroughly into involved skin once to three times daily.

Warts   Salicylic Acid
                 Benzoic Acid $\overline{aa}$ 10
                 Flexible Collodion QS

Paint warts three times a day. Cover with adhesive tape each time.

Index